T0292623

Springer Theses

Recognizing Outstanding Ph.D. Research

Aims and Scope

The series "Springer Theses" brings together a selection of the very best Ph.D. theses from around the world and across the physical sciences. Nominated and endorsed by two recognized specialists, each published volume has been selected for its scientific excellence and the high impact of its contents for the pertinent field of research. For greater accessibility to non-specialists, the published versions include an extended introduction, as well as a foreword by the student's supervisor explaining the special relevance of the work for the field. As a whole, the series will provide a valuable resource both for newcomers to the research fields described, and for other scientists seeking detailed background information on special questions. Finally, it provides an accredited documentation of the valuable contributions made by today's younger generation of scientists.

Theses are accepted into the series by invited nomination only and must fulfill all of the following criteria

- They must be written in good English.
- The topic should fall within the confines of Chemistry, Physics, Earth Sciences, Engineering and related interdisciplinary fields such as Materials, Nanoscience, Chemical Engineering, Complex Systems and Biophysics.
- The work reported in the thesis must represent a significant scientific advance.
- If the thesis includes previously published material, permission to reproduce this must be gained from the respective copyright holder.
- They must have been examined and passed during the 12 months prior to nomination.
- Each thesis should include a foreword by the supervisor outlining the significance of its content.
- The theses should have a clearly defined structure including an introduction accessible to scientists not expert in that particular field.

More information about this series at http://www.springer.com/series/8790

Loris Fichera

Cognitive Supervision for Robot-Assisted Minimally Invasive Laser Surgery

Doctoral Thesis accepted by
the University of Genoa, Italy

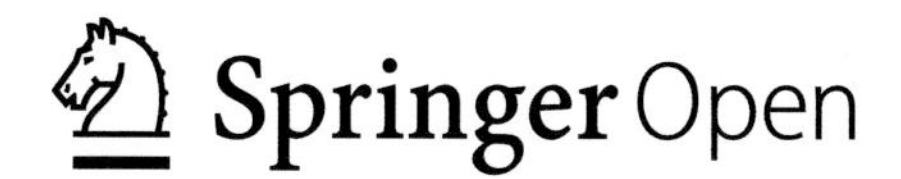

Author
Dr. Loris Fichera
Department of Informatics, Bioengineering, Robotics and Systems Engineering
University of Genoa
Genoa
Italy

and

Department of Advanced Robotics
Istituto Italiano di Tecnologia
Genoa
Italy

Supervisors
Dr. Diego Pardo
Agile and Dexterous Robotics Laboratory
Eidgenössische Technische Hochschule (ETHZ)
Zürich
Switzerland

Dr. Leonardo Serra Mattos
Department of Advanced Robotics
Istituto Italiano di Tecnologia
Genoa
Italy

Prof. Darwin Caldwell
Department of Advanced Robotics
Istituto Italiano di Tecnologia
Genoa
Italy

ISSN 2190-5053 ISSN 2190-5061 (electronic)
Springer Theses
ISBN 978-3-319-30329-1 ISBN 978-3-319-30330-7 (eBook)
DOI 10.1007/978-3-319-30330-7

Library of Congress Control Number: 2016932505

Printed on acid-free paper

This Springer imprint is published by Springer Nature
The registered company is Springer International Publishing AG Switzerland

Parts of this thesis have been published in the following documents:

Journal Publications

L. Fichera, D. Pardo, P. Illiano, D.G. Caldwell, and L.S. Mattos, "On-line Estimation of Laser Incision Depth for Transoral Microsurgery: Approach and Preliminary Evaluation," *The International Journal of Medical Robotics and Computer Assisted Surgery*, [Online]. Available: http://dx.doi.org/10.1002/rcs.1656

D. Pardo, L. Fichera, D.G. Caldwell, and L.S. Mattos, "Learning Temperature Dynamics on Agar-Based Phantom Tissue Surface During Single Point CO2 Laser Exposure," *Neural Processing Letters, vol. 42, no. 1, pp. 55–70, 2015.*

Conference Proceedings

L. Fichera, D. Pardo, P. Illiano, D.G. Caldwell, and L.S. Mattos, "Feed-Forward Incision Control for Laser Microsurgery of Soft Tissue", in *Robotics and Automation (ICRA), 2015 IEEE International Conference on*, pp. 1235–1240, 26–30 May 2015.

D. Pardo, L. Fichera, D.G. Caldwell, and L.S. Mattos, "Thermal Supervision During Robotic Laser Microsurgery", in *Biomedical Robotics and Biomechatronics (Biorob), 2014 5th IEEE RAS & EMBS International Conference on*, pp. 363–368, 12–15 Aug. 2014.

L. Fichera, D. Pardo, and L.S. Mattos, "Supervisory System for Laser-Assisted Phonomicrosurgery", in *Engineering in Medicine and Biology Society (EMBC), 2013 35th Annual International Conference of the IEEE*, pp. 4839–4842, 3–7 July 2013.

L. Fichera, D. Pardo, L.S. Mattos, "Modeling Tissue Temperature Dynamics during Laser Exposure", in *Advances in computational intelligence (IWANN13)*, vol. 7903. Springer, Berlin Heidelberg 2013.

Workshop Abstracts

L. Fichera, D. Pardo, D.G. Caldwell and L.S. Mattos, "New Assistive Technologies for Laser Microsurgery", *4th Joint Workshop on New Technologies for Computer/Robot Assisted Surgery (CRAS)*, Genova, Italy. Oct. 2014.

L. Fichera, D. Pardo, N. Deshpande, and L.S. Mattos, "On-line estimation of ablation depth during CO2-laser exposure", *Workshop on Cognitive Surgical Robotics, IEEE/RSJ IROS 2013*. Tokyo, Japan. November 2013.

L. Fichera, D. Pardo, and L.S. Mattos, "Virtual Supervision for a Virtual Scalpel", *μRALP Workshop, 1st Russian-German Conference on Biomedical Engineering (RCG)*, Hannover, Germany. October 2013.

L. Fichera, D. Pardo and L.S. Mattos, "Artificial Cognitive Supervision during Robot-Assisted Laser Surgery", *3rd Joint Workshop on New Technologies for Computer/Robot Assisted Surgery (CRAS)*, Verona, Italy. September 2013.

Reality is frequently inaccurate.

—Douglas N. Adams

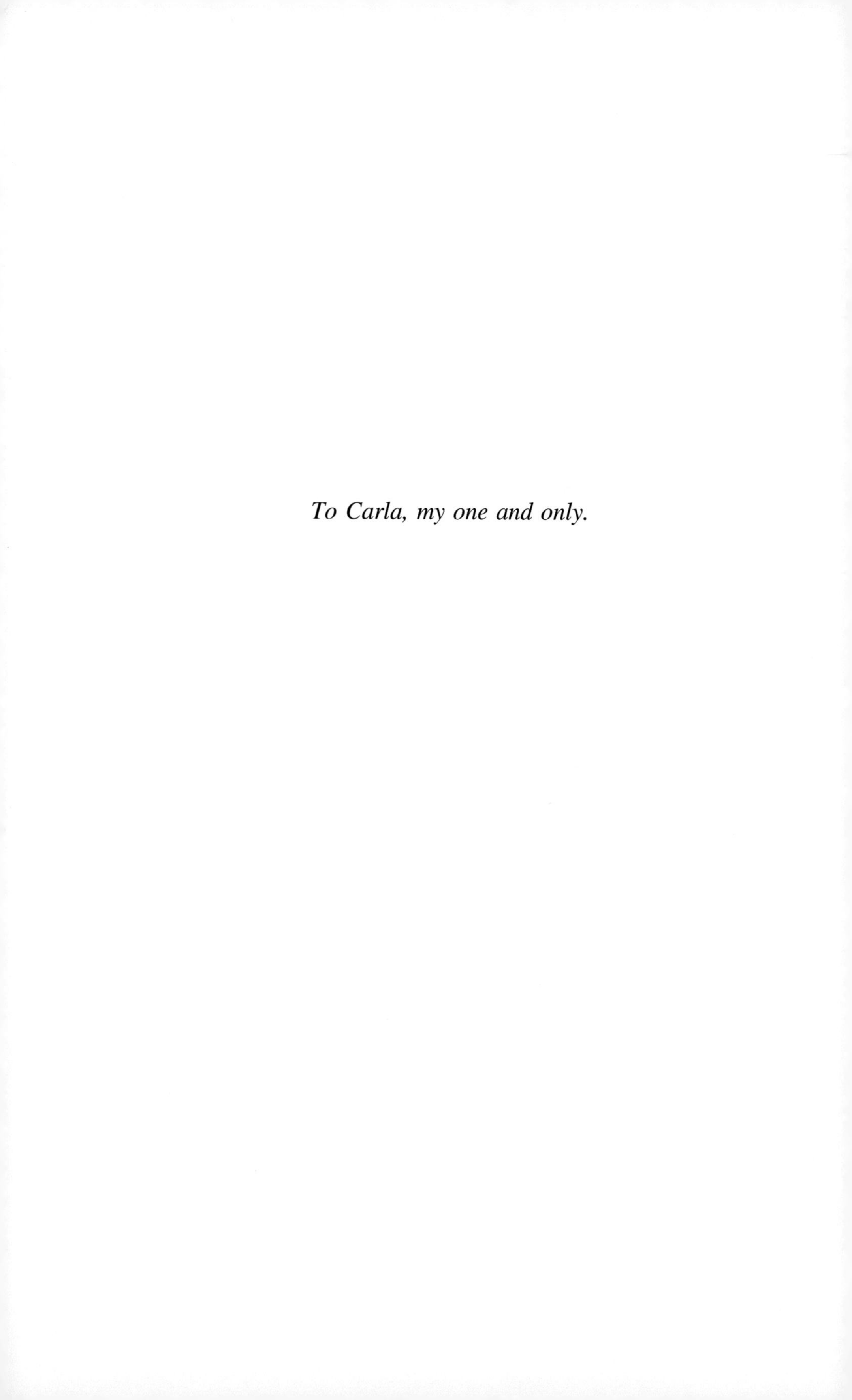

To Carla, my one and only.

Supervisors' Foreword

It is our great pleasure to introduce Dr. Loris Fichera's thesis work, conducted within the Biomedical Robotics Laboratory at the Italian Institute of Technology (IIT). Dr. Fichera started his doctoral study in January 2012 having received a three-year fellowship from IIT to support research within the European Union sponsored project μRALP (Micro-Technologies and Systems for Robot-Assisted Laser Phonomicrosurgery). This project was being coordinated by IIT. The research within this Ph.D. centered on a challenging work package dedicated to the creation of Cognitive Supervisory Systems that would increase surgical performance and safety during robot-assisted laser procedures. Dr. Fichera successfully completed his doctoral study with a final viva voce defense on April 22, 2015, obtaining an excellent (highest) rating.

Dr. Fichera's dissertation presents significant advances to the state of the art in assisted technologies for precise laser surgery of soft tissue. This is an extremely timely contribution as many aspects of modern medicine rely increasingly on lasers for the treatment of pathologies throughout the human body. Laser application areas range from dermatology and dentistry to ophthalmology, gynecology, and neurology. In many of these cases, lasers are used as a precision tool to perform delicate ablation or cutting procedures. One such example is the use of CO_2 lasers in laryngeal microsurgeries, which typically involve highly delicate and complex surgical techniques that have the double aim of treating abnormalities, while preserving as much as possible of the organ functionalities (such as deglutition and voice production). The achievement of these goals often requires a level of precision that is at the limits of (or exceeds) unaided human abilities. It is at these extreme performance limits that the assistive technology work reported by Dr. Fichera's in this thesis has the greatest impact.

During laser surgeries, surgeons face fundamental challenges related to the control of the laser ablation process. This control is vital for a good quality surgical outcome as it dictates the resulting tissue characteristics after the laser irradiation. The creation of precise and high-quality laser incisions requires that the surgeon has an intrinsic understanding of, and feeling for, the energy-based phenomena underlying laser ablation, and the capability to discern and quantify the effects induced by the laser on the tissue, even though these are difficult to perceive. This dissertation presents a number of new approaches to automatically supervise, predict, and control the laser incision/ablation process. This is subsequently shown to enable significant enhancements to the surgical situational awareness, complementing the surgeon's perception of the state of the target tissue and facilitating precise incision control.

In this work, Dr. Fichera reformulates the laser ablation modeling problem using a cognitive systems approach. Machine learning methods are investigated and used to reach this goal, inspired by the capability of experienced surgeons to achieve precise and clean laser cutting. More specifically, the problem is formulated as the estimation of variables that are representative of the state of the tissue during laser cutting, leading to the development of models able to accurately predict tissue surface temperature and laser incision depth. These are highly relevant parameters for soft tissue laser surgery as they allow enhanced controllability and minimize thermal damage in the surgical area, leading to improved surgical precision and quality.

The results presented in this dissertation are based on meticulous experimental work conducted by Dr. Fichera in collaboration with surgeons and microscopy experts. A large amount of data was collected during carefully planned laser–tissue interaction experiments, providing a wealth of information for the modeling process and for the validation of the approach. Furthermore, user (including clinician) trials with the proposed technology integrated into a robot-assisted laser microsurgery system demonstrated its suitability for real-time applications and its applicability to real surgical scenarios. This successful testing is a further endorsement of the significance of the technological achievement, when compared against the current state of the art, which uses numerical computation methods that have a high computational cost and are not straightforward to implement in a surgical setting.

Genoa, Italy
November 2015

Dr. Diego Pardo
Dr. Leonardo Serra Mattos
Prof. Darwin Caldwell

Acknowledgments

From the most profound depths of my heart, I am grateful to those who have supported me throughout these years of doctoral studies.

First and foremost, I thank Dr. Leonardo Mattos for having accepted me into the Laboratory of Biomedical Robotics at the Istituto Italiano di Tecnologia, and for proposing me to be part of the µRALP project. His trust and confidence were most essential in keeping my motivation high as I progressed through the various stages of the Ph.D. program. He has been a continual source of inspiration to me, and I could only hope that I have inherited a portion of his commitment and enthusiasm.

I thank Prof. Darwin Caldwell for giving me the opportunity to work in the Department of Advanced Robotics, for his interest, support, and invaluable feedback.

This Ph.D. is owed to my close collaboration with Dr. Diego Pardo, with whom I formed the "µRALP Work Package 10" team, and whose patience and relentless efforts have forged me ahead. Thank you for instilling in me your passion for research, and for the time and energy you spent in helping me find my research direction. Also, for having reviewed dozens of my written drafts!

I am very grateful to the clinical staff and research team of the Department of Otolaryngology at the San Martino University Hospital: Prof. Giorgio Peretti, Dr. Francesco Mora and Dr. Luca Guastini. They have introduced me to the medical background necessary for my research, and provided crucial inputs and comments. I owe a big debt of gratitude to my friend and fellow student Placido Illiano, who has taught me the tissue manipulation and analysis techniques used throughout this dissertation. His technical inputs were most instrumental in the making of this research. I shall always remember his positive attitude every time I came with a new idea: "We can do this, let's discuss this over a coffee!" Besides being a talented researcher, Placido is a cherished friend with whom I shared the many ups and downs of Ph.D. life.

In the course of my doctoral studies, I was blessed with meeting two wonderful people who have deeply influenced my personal and intellectual development: Dr. Joshua Schultz and Dr. Nikhil Deshpande. The long discussions we had, on topics ranging from linguistics to life choices, have had a great impact on me and contributed to my own thinking. I am grateful that they shared their experience and wisdom with me, while I was going through this grand challenge.

This thesis could have not come to fruition without the encouragements, suggestions, and tips of several colleagues (past and present) at IIT: Minh Ha Quang, Giulio Dagnino, Marco San Biagio, Agnese Abrusci, Adrian Ramos Peon, Veronica Penza, Emidio Olivieri, Manish Chauhan, Giacinto Barresi, Alperen Acemoğlu, Lucia Schiatti, Cheng Zhuoqi, Erica Barini, Stefano Toxiri, Matteo Russo, Federico Tinarelli, Edoardo Balzani, Francesco Asta. Thank you for all you did. A special call-out to Jesus Ortiz, whose technical skills, smart thinking, and humility I admire greatly.

I must express my appreciation to the dedicated supporting staff at IIT: Valentina Rosso, Simona Ventriglia, Monica Vasco, Floriana Sardi, Simona Montana, Elisa Repetti, Riccardo Sepe, Gianluca Pane, Giuseppe Sofia, Marco Migliorini, Nick Dring. Special thanks to Silvia Ivaldi for having helped me to unravel the many arcane mysteries of the Travel Expense Management software.

Thank you to my flatmates (and fellow Ph.D. students) Davide De Tommaso and Bilal Ur Rehman for their sincere friendship, and for having shared the marvelous view of Genova from our terrace all these nights!

I would like to acknowledge the singular contribution of my bass guitar teacher, Francesco Olivieri. Learning the bass has been such a release for me during the hard times of the Ph.D., and has become an irreplaceable component of my life. Ultimately, I shall aspire to be able to play the most difficult key, that is, the *key of life*.

I am profoundly grateful to all of the teachers and mentors who have helped me on my educational—and life—path, from primary school through graduate school. Thank you all.

To my big family, for a lifetime of love and support. Especially to my uncle Gianni, who prematurely passed away in 2014. He introduced me to the many secrets of Genova when I first arrived in 2011, and we shared the same passion for this city.

Finally, I owe a unique debt of gratitude to my beautiful wife Carla. Her love, patience, and grace flow more abundantly than I deserve. God only knows what I would be without her.

The research leading to these results has received funding from the European Union Seventh Framework Programme FP7/2007–2013—Challenge 2—Cognitive Systems, Interaction, Robotics—under grant agreement μRALP No. 288233.

Contents

About the Author

Loris Fichera was born in Vittoria, a lively town located in southeastern Sicily, at the very center of the Mediterranean. Since his teen years, he got the opportunity to travel, visiting several countries across Europe and beyond. Loris attended the Liceo Scientifico Cannizzaro in Vittoria and later enrolled in the Computer Engineering program at the University of Catania. He graduated in 2008 with a Bachelor's degree and in 2011 with a Master's degree, both Cum Laude. From 2008 to 2011, he was a member of the Eurobot UNICT Team at the University of Catania, where he moved his first steps in the field of Robotics. As a member of the team, he took part in the *Eurobot Open* Robotics competition—being a runner-up in the 2009 and 2011 editions. In 2010, he was a visiting research fellow at the University of Hertfordshire, United Kingdom, supported by an Erasmus Placement Mobility Grant. Driven by the curiosity to pursue deeper knowledge in the field of Robotics, he joined the Department of Advanced Robotics at the Istituto Italiano di Tecnologia as a Ph.D. student in January 2012. From 2012 to 2015 he has been a contributor to the European project µRALP, focusing on the development of new technologies for robot-assisted laser microsurgery. He is currently a Postdoctoral Research Scholar at Vanderbilt University, Tennessee, United States.

Chapter 1
Introduction

Lasers constitute a versatile tool in the treatment of diverse pathologies affecting delicate and vital human organs. Transoral laser microsurgery (TLM) is one important field of application. This is a suite of minimally invasive endoscopic techniques for the excision of minuscule laryngeal abnormalities [1, 2]. In these procedures, lasers are utilized for a variety of tasks, including precise tissue cutting, ablation and coagulation. The advantage over traditional cold instrument surgery is manifold: the combination of high power and minute beam focusing (down to a few hundreds microns in diameter) allows for the creation of small, clean incisions through tissues [1]. Lasers present the unique advantage of being able to cut and coagulate tissues at the same time, thus offering an enhanced control of bleeding [1, 2]. Laser cutting facilitates the cicatrizazion of tissues, resulting in less post-operative complications and shorter patient recovery time [2, 3]. Additional benefits of laser microsurgery in the larynx over other treatment modalities include smaller cost-per-procedure [4] and lower postoperative morbidity [1, 3].

Despite these many advantages, the use of the laser as surgical tool is not straightforward. To qualify for TLM, clinicians are required to undertake specialized training, aimed at developing a safe and effective laser cutting technique [2, 5]. In the surgical equipment available today, laser control consists of two parts:

- **Control of Laser Positioning**, which is required to delineate and execute the desired incision lines on tissues. In TLM, the laser position is controlled manually through a mechanical device called laser micromanipulator [6]. Because of the minuscule size of the organs involved, these interventions are carried out under microscope magnification. The micromanipulator is an effective control interface, yet it is difficult to master, especially because it breaks the hand-eye coordination of the operator [7].

L. Fichera, *Cognitive Supervision for Robot-Assisted Minimally Invasive Laser Surgery*, Springer Theses, DOI 10.1007/978-3-319-30330-7_1

- **Control of the Laser Parameters**, these determine the characteristics of the resulting incision, i.e. depth, width and thermal effects on surrounding tissues. Modern laser systems such as the Lumenis Ultrapulse® or the Deka SmartXide[2] ENT present diverse parameters—including output power, spot size, pulse frequency and duration, exposure time. In the course of an intervention, these parameters are adjusted depending on the operative task at hand. For each application, no fixed set of parameters exists: clinicians may use different settings, depending on their skills, experience and preferred technique [1].

Evidently, laser microsurgeries require clinicians to possess a strong dexterity in the use of the laser for the management of soft tissues. The limitations mentioned above have recently stimulated new research and technological developments in this area: numerous works have explored the creation of computer/robot-assisted laser microsurgery systems [6–14], aimed to allow clinicians to control the laser motion through a digital computer and a robotic device. Support is provided for motion scaling, as well as for the automatic execution of pre-planned motion patterns, that enhance the precision and safety of laser microsurgery.

While recent developments have facilitated precise laser motions, the automatic control of laser incisions has not been realized until now, and remains largely unexplored. It is not evident how to regulate the laser operational parameters in order to achieve high quality incisions: this would require modeling the physical interactions that occur between laser light and tissue, which are inherently complex and not straightforward to describe [15, 16]. The control of laser incisions is performed manually by clinicians, who need to complete extensive practice to learn how laser parameters influence the laser cutting process. Learning the association between the manipulation of laser parameters and the corresponding effects on tissues is not straightforward, and is regarded as an essential component of a laser surgeon's skills set [2, 4, 5, 17]. Based on these challenges, the subject of this thesis is to lay out the groundwork for the monitoring and control of laser incisions during microsurgeries.

Laser incision of soft tissues is understood as an energy-based, thermal process: the energy associated with the laser beam is absorbed by the tissue under the form of heat, producing a local rise of temperature. Continuous temperature increase eventually breaks molecular bonds and results in the ejection of hot plume. This process is commonly referred to as *thermal laser ablation* and has been extensively studied in the past [15, 16], but has never been modeled for monitoring or control purposes. In this thesis, we build models capable of describing the development of laser incisions in soft tissues, given the same inputs used by the clinicians, i.e. the laser operational parameters.

Recent years have seen a growing interest in the use of artificial cognitive systems to monitor and control complex processes, that would be difficult to manage using classic control methods [18]. In the scope of this doctoral dissertation, we view artificial cognition as the framework of choice to model specific laser-induced effects on tissues, and use these models to endow surgical laser systems with the capacity to both monitor and the control such effects.

1.1 Motivations

This section presents an example that provides a qualitative description of the problems that motivate the research described in this dissertation. Figure 1.1 shows a magnified view of the human vocal folds, on which a tumor is highlighted. This is a Squamous Cell Carcinoma (SCC) [19], a common type of laryngeal cancer whose occurrence is primarily related to smoke and alcohol consumption [20]. SCC originates from the cells that constitute the superficial layers of the epithelium and may spread to contiguous structures [21], potentially impairing phonatory abilities. In addition to this, laryngeal SCC is a life-threatening disease: it is estimated that nearly 20 000 Europeans died of laryngeal cancer in 2012 [22].

When treating malignancies of the vocal folds, it is important not just to eradicate the tumor, but also to preserve as much organ functionality as possible. In practice, this translates to the use of surgical strategies aimed to minimize the extent of the dissection. Given the small size of the vocal folds, these interventions require greater precision: even 1 m of additionally resected tissue can make the difference between a successful resection and permanent vocal impairment [23, 24]. In this respect, the ability to control the depth of laser incisions is of paramount importance. This is influenced not just by the parameters that characterize the laser irradiation—such as laser power and exposure time—but also by the type and molecular composition of tissue, which is inherently inhomogeneous [25]. The laser incision depth decided *a priori* might not correspond to the actual one, therefore this must be tracked to ensure appropriate results. The contactless cutting method of the laser prevents clinicians from using their delicate sense of touch to discern the actual depth of incision, thus visual inspection is the only tool available to interpret the laser penetration depth.

Another factor of risk for the vocal function is represented by the onset of collateral laser-induced effects. Laser cutting of soft tissues is a thermal process, whose consequences might include not just the desired dissection, but also permanent tissue damage. Carbonization, for instance, occurs when the tissue temperature rises above 100 °C, typically in the surroundings of the incision line [15]. It commonly occurs because of an erroneous selection of laser parameters, e.g. long laser exposure, and results in non-intentional damage of healthy tissues that should have been preserved.

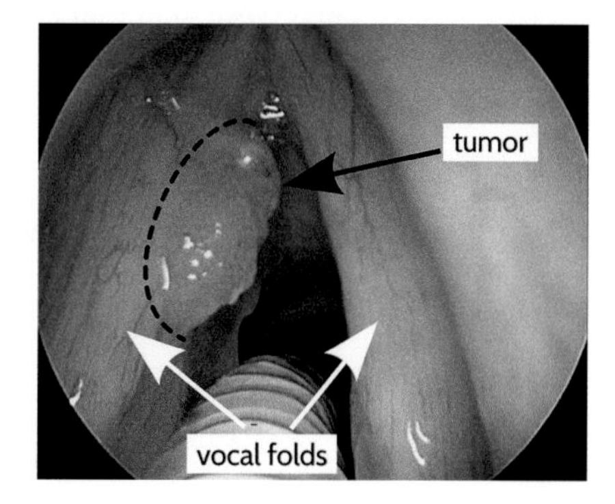

Fig. 1.1 Squamous cell carcinoma of the vocal folds. Image courtesy of Prof. Giorgio Peretti, MD, Clinica Otorinolaringoiatrica, Università di Genova

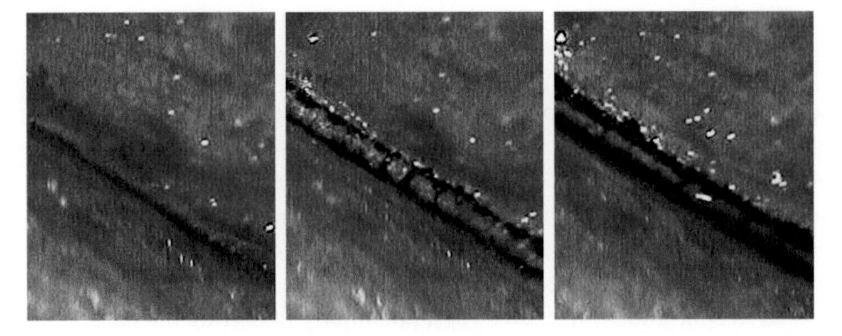

Fig. 1.2 Sequence showing progressive carbonization of soft tissue during interaction with CO_2 laser radiation. Reproduced from [26] with kind permission from Springer Science+Business Media

The onset of carbonization is not easy to control, as it offers limited visual cues: the tissue blackening associated with it (Fig. 1.2) appears once damage has already occurred. To optimize medical outcomes, carbonization should be avoided [15], as it leads to a longer patient healing time and may leave scars, diminishing the quality of surgery [27].

From the simple scenario described above, it is apparent that the control of the incision process relies entirely on the experience and dexterity of the surgeon, who intrinsically establishes the state of the cutting and thereby decides the laser actions to be perform. The interaction between the laser and the tissue is the elemental building block at the core of laser-based surgery: it is through this interaction that incisions are performed. Unfortunately, nowadays there are no technical solutions for the automatic supervision of this process. To this end, a predictive model would be necessary, i.e. a model that allows to predict the outcome of the laser-tissue interaction process is needed. Analytical models of laser-tissue interactions (LTI) are well known [15]: these seem impractical to use in our scenario, as they admit a solution only under very strict assumptions. Furthermore, these models depend on a considerable number of variables representing properties of both the laser and the tissue (e.g. laser wavelength, absorption and scattering coefficients of tissue, tissue thermal conductivity, etc.), that are not straightforward to measure in a surgical setup. If a system is supposed to supervise the state of the LTI, it should rely on inputs similar to those used by surgeons and not on analytical models based on tissue properties. Accordingly, we propose to use models motivated by the capacity of humans to map and fuse diverse sets of information and infer the future state of events.

1.2 Components of the Research

This doctoral dissertation develops at the intersection of three distinct fields of research, as illustrated in Fig. 1.3. The work described here is part of a larger research effort, called the μRALP project [28]. This EU-funded project proposes to redesign and improve the state-of-the-art setup for laser microsurgeries. Through research and development in a range of topics including human-machine interfaces, assistive

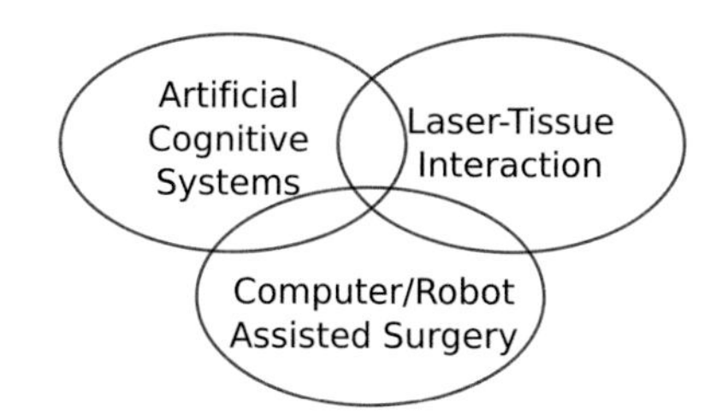

Fig. 1.3 The research presented in this dissertation resides at the intersection of different fields

systems, medical imaging, endoscopic tools, and micromanipulators the project aims to improve the levels of accessibility, precision and safety in this kind of procedures. The ultimate goal is the creation of an advanced surgical robotic platform, enabling surgeons to perform operations that would not be possible using the current technology. The μRALP platform aims to enhance the surgeon's perception of the surgical site and support his decision-making process by means of an information-rich interface based on augmented reality.

In the scope of the μRALP project, the objective of this research is establish the ground for the development of novel technologies for computer-assisted laser surgery. These shall provide the clinician with support for the automatic control/monitoring of laser incisions during microsurgeries. To enable these technologies, here we conduct an investigation of the laser ablation process, and derive models capable of mapping the application of laser light to its corresponding effects on tissue. It is important to point out that the objective of our modeling is not to describe the physical interactions between laser light and tissues. Rather, we shall focus on the analysis and synthesis of higher-level effects, which are relevant from a clinical point of view.

The use of a forward model to predict the outcomes of the laser ablation process is a problem in which analytical modeling is neither convenient nor viable. For this reason, here we explore *cognitive* models, i.e. models that attempt to replicate human cognitive processes for the purpose of predicting the future state of events. Specifically, we develop models of the laser incision process based on the same high-level information used by the surgeons: laser activation, power, pulse duration and exposure time. These models are extracted through the use of statistical learning techniques from data collected during controlled laser experiments.

1.3 Scope of the Thesis

The main contribution of this thesis is the application of a statistical learning approach to infer models of LTI that are straightforward to use in a surgical setup, and which enable enhanced precision in laser-based surgical operations.

1. A model for the estimation of the tissue temperature during laser ablation is derived. The model extends current analytic models in that it accounts for temperature variation induced by a moving laser beam.
2. A model for the estimation of the laser cutting depth during laser incision is extracted. The obtained model extends the scope of application of a similar class of

solutions (steady state models [16]), demonstrating their feasibility for laryngeal laser microsurgery.
3. The inverse model for the laser cutting depth enables different strategies for the controlled ablation of soft tissues. Here we present and validate one such strategy by demonstrating automatic control of laser incision depth on soft tissue.
4. The models of LTI enable the supervision of the laser cutting process, thus enabling the development of practical technologies that assist and guide clinicians during laser microsurgery.

1.4 Outline of the Thesis

This dissertation is articulated into seven chapters, the remaining of which are organized as follows:

Chapter 2 presents the theoretical background of this dissertation. The fundamentals of laser technology and laser-matter interactions are introduced. Particular focus is given to the mechanisms of thermal laser ablation of biological tissues. The equations governing these processes are reviewed and discussed.

Chapter 3 introduces the research questions that motivate the research described in this dissertation. These are related to the use of statistical learning theory to model the laser incision of soft tissues. Materials and methods employed in our investigation are presented here.

Chapter 4 presents a novel methodology to model tissue temperature dynamics during laser incision. This process is modeled through the superposition of Gaussian basis functions, whose parameters are estimated through a nonlinear fitting technique.

Chapter 5 presents a novel approach to estimate the laser cutting depth in soft tissues. A simple linear regression is demonstrated to provide sufficient modeling accuracy for surgical applications of lasers. The inverse model is used to enable the controlled laser ablation of soft tissues.

Chapter 6 presents a practical implementation of the models derived in the previous chapters. This chapter demonstrates the concept of a system capable of monitoring the laser incision process in a real operating scenario.

Chapter 7 concludes this dissertation and provides some suggestions regarding future directions of research related to this work.

References

1. M. Rubinstein, W. Armstrong, Transoral laser microsurgery for laryngeal cancer: a primer and review of laser dosimetry. Lasers Med. Sci. **26**(1), 113–124 (2011)
2. V. Oswal, M. Remacle, Transoral laser laryngeal surgery, in *Principles and Practice of Lasers in Otorhinolaryngology and Head and Neck*, 2nd edn., ed. by O. Vasant, R. Marc (Kugler Publications, Amsterdam, The Netherlands, 2014), pp. 99–116
3. G. Peretti, C. Piazza, F. Del Bon, R. Mora, P. Grazioli, D. Barbieri, S. Mangili, P. Nicolai, Function preservation using transoral laser surgery for T2–T3 glottic cancer: oncologic, vocal, and swallowing outcomes. Eur. Arch. Otorhinolaryngol. Official J. Eur. Fed. Otorhinolaryngol. Soc. (EUFOS) **270**(8), 2275–2281 (2013)
4. H. Sims, T. Brennan, Laser treatment for head and neck cancer, in *Head & Neck Cancer: Current Perspectives, Advances, and Challenges*, ed. by J.A. Radosevich (Springer, Netherlands, 2013), pp. 621–648
5. W. Steiner, P. Ambrosch, Endoscopic laser surgery of the upper aerodigestive tract: with special emphasis on cancer surgery. Thieme (2000)
6. M. Remacle, G. Lawson, M.-C. Nollevaux, M. Delos, Current state of scanning micromanipulator applications with the carbon dioxide laser. Ann. Otol. Rhinol. Laryngol. **117**(4), 239–244 (2008)
7. N. Deshpande, J. Ortiz, D. Caldwell, L. Mattos, Enhanced computer-assisted laser microsurgeries with a "virtual microscope" based surgical system, in *IEEE International Conference on Robotics and Automation (ICRA)*, 2014, May 2014, pp. 4194–4199
8. L.S. Mattos, N. Deshpande, G. Barresi, L. Guastini, G. Peretti, A novel computerized surgeon machine interface for robot-assisted laser phonomicrosurgery. The Laryngoscope **124**(8), 1887–1894 (2014)
9. Y.-T. Wong, C.C. Finley, J.F. Giallo, R.A. Buckmire, Novel co2 laser robotic controller outperforms experienced laser operators in tasks of accuracy and performance repeatability. The Laryngoscope **121**(8), 1738–1742 (2011)
10. H.-W. Tang, H.V. Brussel, J.V. Sloten, D. Reynaerts, G. De Win, B.V. Cleynenbreugel, P.R. Koninckx, Evaluation of an intuitive writing interface in robot-aided laser laparoscopic surgery. Comput. Aided Surg. **11**(1), 21–30 (2006)
11. M. Remacle, F. Hassan, D. Cohen, G. Lawson, M. Delos, New computer-guided scanner for improving co2 laser-assisted microincision. Eur. Arch. Otorhinolaryngol. Head & Neck **262**(2), 113–119 (2005)
12. J.F. Giallo, A medical robotic system for laser phonomicrosurgery. Ph.D. dissertation, North Carolina State University (2008)
13. L. Mattos, G. Dagnino, G. Becattini, M. Dellepiane, D. Caldwell, A virtual scalpel system for computer-assisted laser microsurgery, in *2011 IEEE/RSJ International Conference on Intelligent Robots and Systems (IROS)* vol. 2011, pp. 1359–1365
14. S.C. Desai, C.-K. Sung, D.W. Jang, E.M. Genden, Transoral robotic surgery using a carbon dioxide flexible laser for tumors of the upper aerodigestive tract. The Laryngoscope **118**(12), 2187–2189 (2008)
15. M. Niemz, *Laser-tissue Interactions* (Springer, Berlin Heidelberg, 2004)
16. A. Vogel, V. Venugopalan, Mechanisms of pulsed laser ablation of biological tissues. Chem. Rev. **103**(2), 577–644 (2003)
17. Y. Yan, A.E. Olszewski, M.R. Hoffman, P. Zhuang, C.N. Ford, S.H. Dailey, J.J. Jiang, Use of lasers in laryngeal surgery. J. Voice **24**(1), 102–109 (2010)

18. Ict—Information and Communication Technologies. work programme 2011–2012. http://cordis.europa.eu/fp7/ict/components/documents/ict-wp-2011-12-en.pdf. Accessed on 03 Mar 2015 (Online)
19. L. Barnes, L. Tse, J. Hunt, M. Brandwein-Gensler, M. Urken, P. Slootweg, N. Gale, A. Cardesa, N. Zidar, P. Boffetta, Tumours of the hypopharynx, larynx and trachea: Introduction, ed. by L. Barnes, J. Eveson, P. Reichart, D. Sidransky, in *World Health Organization Classification of Tumours Pathology and Genetics of Head and Neck Tumours* (IARC Press, Lyon, 2005), pp. 111–117
20. A. Altieri, W. Garavello, C. Bosetti, S. Gallus, C.L. Vecchia, Alcohol consumption and risk of laryngeal cancer. Oral Oncol. **41**(10), 956–965 (2005)
21. J.A. Kirchner, Two hundred laryngeal cancers: patterns of growth and spread as seen in serial section. The Laryngoscope **87**(4), 474–482 (1977)
22. J. Ferlay, E. Steliarova-Foucher, J. Lortet-Tieulent, S. Rosso, J. Coebergh, H. Comber, D. Forman, F. Bray, Cancer incidence and mortality patterns in europe: estimates for 40 countries in 2012. Eur. J. Cancer **49**(6), 1374–1403 (2013)
23. M.L. Hinni, A. Ferlito, M.S. Brandwein-Gensler, R.P. Takes, C.E. Silver, W.H. Westra, R.R. Seethala, J.P. Rodrigo, J. Corry, C.R. Bradford, J.L. Hunt, P. Strojan, K.O. Devaney, D.R. Gnepp, D.M. Hartl, L.P. Kowalski, A. Rinaldo, L. Barnes, Surgical margins in head and neck cancer: a contemporary review. Head Neck **35**(9), 1362–1370 (2013)
24. M. Alicandri-Ciufelli, M. Bonali, A. Piccinini, L. Marra, A. Ghidini, E. Cunsolo, A. Maiorana, L. Presutti, P. Conte, Surgical margins in head and neck squamous cell carcinoma: what is close? Eur. Arch. Otorhinolaryngol. **270**(10), 2603–2609 (2013)
25. S.L. Jacques, Optical properties of biological tissues: a review. Phys. Med. Biol. **58**(11), R37 (2013)
26. D. Pardo, L. Fichera, D. Caldwell, L. Mattos, Learning temperature dynamics on agar-based phantom tissue surface during single point co2 laser exposure. Neural Process. Lett. **42**(1), 55–70 (2015). http://dx.doi.org/10.1007/s11063-014-9389-y (Online)
27. R. Steiner, Laser-tissue interactions, in *Laser and IPL Technology in Dermatology and Aesthetic Medicine*, ed. by C. Raulin, S. Karsai (Springer, Berlin, 2011), pp. 23–36
28. The microralp project, http://www.microralp.eu. Accessed 03 Mar 2015 (Online)

Chapter 2
Background: Laser Technology and Applications to Clinical Surgery

The goal of this chapter is to provide the background that frames the research described in this dissertation. Principles and concepts relevant to the content of subsequent chapters are introduced here. Because this work resides at the intersection of laser-tissue interaction with computer-assisted surgery, the basics of laser technology are introduced here.

Modern surgical laser systems are advanced instruments whose functioning is based on technology derived from a variety of different disciplines, including optics, electromagnetism, electronics. Rather than describing the composition of a modern laser system in detail, here we present a generic description of the mechanisms that permit the generation of laser light. In laser surgery, laser beams are primarily used as scalpels, i.e. as tools to perform incisions and resections. Laser-induced effects on tissue are manifold; although some of them are advantageous, others can produce irreparable damage and diminish the overall quality of surgery. Here, we review these effects and explain how they can be generated and controlled.

The chapter starts with an overview of the physical phenomena that are exploited in the generation of laser light. An understanding of these phenomena is an essential prerequisite to understand the variety of laser sources available today: these are classified primarily by their wavelength, intensity and spot size. The properties of laser light will be described and contrasted with the characteristics of light produced by traditional incandescent sources. Laser sources produce highly intense beams of nearly monochromatic light, which are known to produce numerous interesting effects on the material they traverse. These effects will be discussed in the latter part of the chapter, which focuses on light-matter interactions. A class of interactions will be reviewed in greater detail, namely *thermal interactions*: these are implemented in numerous medical applications for therapeutic purposes. In the context of laser surgery, thermal interactions are used to produce incisions on tissue. The physical processes that enable the creation of laser incisions on biological tissue will be described. Finally, the advantages and shortcomings of laser cutting of tissues will be addressed.

L. Fichera, *Cognitive Supervision for Robot-Assisted Minimally Invasive Laser Surgery*, Springer Theses, DOI 10.1007/978-3-319-30330-7_2

2.1 Physical Properties of Light

Our understanding of the nature of light is based on the fact that it exhibits properties of both electromagnetic (EM) waves and elementary particles, this characteristic is known as the wave-particle duality [1]. First, we consider the description of light as EM waves; the terms *light* and *EM radiation* are used interchangeably throughout this dissertation. Light can be regarded as the perturbation produced by the interplay of mutually related electric and magnetic fields. Each pair of electric/magnetic fields is characterized by a common wavelength λ and oscillate perpendicular with each other and at right angle to the direction of propagation, as shown in Fig. 2.1. In general, EM radiation is classified according to the range of wavelengths it contains. The EM spectrum covers all the possible wavelengths of EM radiation: a limited interval is shown in Fig. 2.2, ranging from longer wavelengths (Microwaves) to shorter (X-Rays). A fundamental physical property of EM waves is the frequency ν, which relates to the wavelength through the relation $c = \nu \cdot \lambda$, where c is the speed of EM waves in vacuum.

The classic picture of light as EM waves can be revisited in the perspective of the quantum theory. In its simplest form, the theory describes light as the

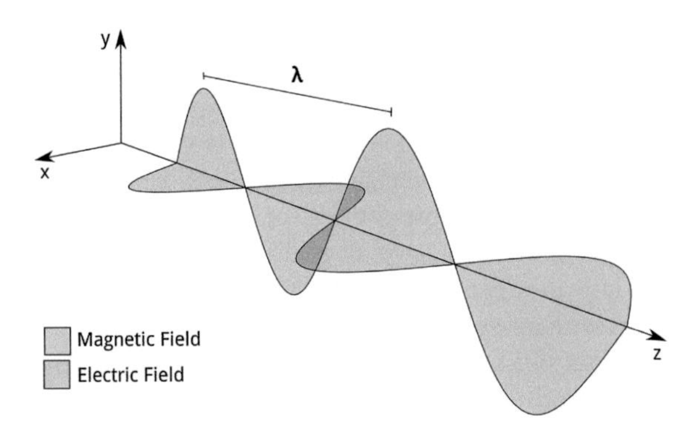

Fig. 2.1 Electromagnetic wave propagating along the z axis of a Cartesian reference frame $Oxyz$. This wave is formed by a pair of mutually related electric and magnetic field, oscillating perpendicular to each other at the same wavelength λ

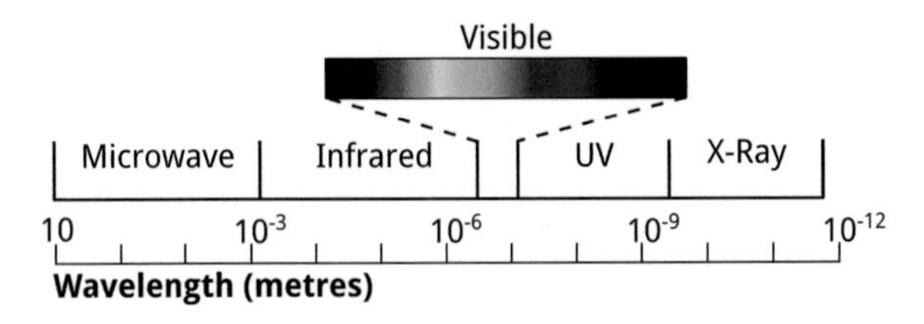

Fig. 2.2 Electromagnetic Spectrum. Note that the relation between wavelength (λ) and frequency (ν) of an electromagnetic wave is $\lambda\nu = c$, where c is the speed of propagation of electromagnetic waves in vacuum

Table 2.1 Radiometric quantities and units used throughout this dissertation

Quantity	Symbol	Unit
Power density, intensity, irradiance	I	$\mathrm{W \cdot m^{-2}}$
Energy density, fluence	E	$\mathrm{J \cdot m^{-2}}$
Volumetric power density	S	$\mathrm{W \cdot m^{-3}}$
Volumetric energy density	E_v	$\mathrm{J \cdot m^{-3}}$

transport of energy through a region of space. The transport is associated with the flow of subatomic particles, called photons, each carrying an energy quantified by $E_{photon} = h\nu$ [1], where ν is the frequency of the electromagnetic wave, as per the EM wave description; h is the Planck's constant.

As we shall see later in this chapter, energy created by a light source can be delivered to matter to alter its physical properties. The interaction of light with matter depends on the amount of energy involved, as well as on the size of the area (or volume) under irradiation. These quantities are often combined into a single radiometric parameter. Different parameters exist, their nomenclature is not uniform throughout the literature. In this dissertation the power density I, the energy density E, the volumetric power density S and the correspondent energy density E_v are most used. For the sake of clarity, Table 2.1 lists these quantities with their units and alternative names they are commonly attributed in the literature.

2.2 Fundamentals of Lasers

Laser stands as an acronym for *Light Amplification by Stimulated Emission of Radiation*. This term identifies the principle of operation of a class of devices that use optical amplification to produce an intense beam of highly directional, monochromatic light [2]. *Stimulated emission* is a physical process that occurs when a medium is exposed to an EM field: light is emitted as a result of the interaction of the field with the atoms of that medium. The emission is characterized by the same wavelength and phase of the incoming radiation. This contrasts with the other known emission process, i.e. *spontaneous emission*: in this case, light propagates in all directions with random wavelength and phase [2]. Spontaneous and stimulated emission are general phenomena that occur naturally at any light source: the intensity of each emission can be characterized by the number of photons that are released. It can be shown that, for a given medium in thermal equilibrium at temperature T, subject to an EM field at frequency ν, the ratio of the photons emitted by spontaneous (P_{sp}) and stimulated emissions (P_{st}) is

$$\frac{P_{sp}}{P_{st}} = \exp\left(\frac{h\nu}{kT}\right) - 1, \tag{2.1}$$

where k is the Boltzmann's constant. This relation establishes the dependency of the light emission with the frequency of the EM field. At frequencies $\nu > kT/h$, spontaneous emission dominates the process: for instance, let us consider the

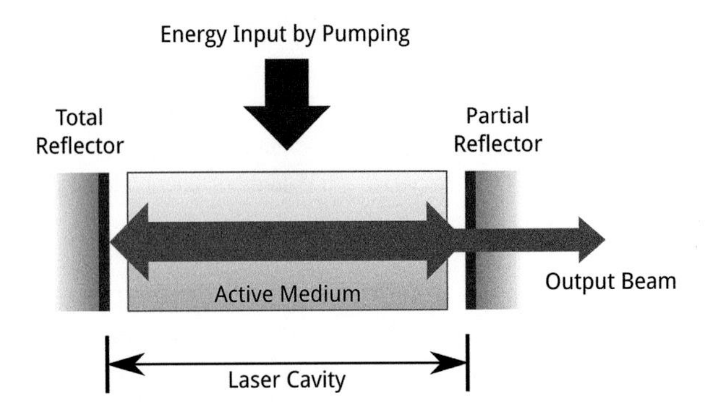

Fig. 2.3 Basic structure of a laser system

filament of a light bulb emitting yellow light ($\nu = 5 \times 10^{14}$ Hz, see Fig. 2.2) at a temperature of $T = 2000$ K, then Eq. 2.1 yields that $P_{sp}/P_{st} \approx 1.5 \times 10^5$. This example is indicative of how the emission of visible traditional light sources consists predominantly of spontaneous emission. Conversely, stimulated emission strongly prevails at long wavelengths, e.g. in the far infrared and microwave ranges. To have significant stimulated emission at wavelengths shorter than far infrared, it is necessary that a particular condition is met, referred to as *population inversion* [2]. This entails altering the distribution of the atomic energy levels in a medium, so that more atoms reside in higher energy states than in the lower. A population inversion can be artificially created pumping energy into the medium, either by means of a traditional powerful light source (optical pumping) or establishing a current flow into it (electrical pumping) [2].

The basic working principle of a laser device is illustrated in Fig. 2.3. A laser system is typically composed of two main parts: (i) a cavity filled with an active medium and (ii) a pump source that injects energy into the medium, thus creating a population inversion that triggers the stimulated emission of light. The cavity is enclosed by two reflective optical elements which force the light to travel back and forth through the medium. Further stimulated emission is produced at each pass, resulting in an optical amplification effect. Once the system has built up a sufficient amount of energy, a fractional part of the light trapped in the cavity escapes through one the reflecting mirrors; this is designed in such a way to have non vanishing transmission at the laser characteristic frequency. The light that escapes the cavity forms the output beam of the laser. Several different materials can be employed as active medium: these include solids, gases, fluids, semiconductors; the choice of the medium determines the wavelength at which stimulated emission occurs.

2.2.1 Laser Beam Optics

The optical properties of a laser beam describe how this propagates through space and the light intensity associated with it. These properties are dictated by the design of the laser device; specifically by the geometry of the cavity and the shape of the mirrors used to confine light into it.

In general, the propagation of light within an homogeneous medium can be formulated in terms of a wave equation, i.e. a second-order partial differential equation that describes how the electric field **E** and the magnetic field **B** associated with the light wave behave in such material. The wave equation is derived from the Maxwell's equations: assuming a medium with relative permeability μ_r $(N \cdot A^{-2})$ and permittivity ε_r $(F \cdot \mathrm{m}^{-1})$, the wave equation takes the form [3]:

$$\nabla^2 \mathbf{E} = \varepsilon_0 \mu_0 \varepsilon_r \mu_r \frac{\partial^2 \mathbf{E}}{\partial t^2},$$
$$\nabla^2 \mathbf{B} = \varepsilon_0 \mu_0 \varepsilon_r \mu_r \frac{\partial^2 \mathbf{B}}{\partial t^2}, \tag{2.2}$$

where μ_0 and ε_0 are the permeability and the permittivity of vacuum, respectively. Equation 2.2 can be solved to obtain a description of the propagation of light which escapes the cavity of a laser device. The form of the solution depends on the specific boundary conditions imposed by the size of the cavity, the shape and type of the reflective optical elements.

Gaussian Beams constitute a set of solutions to Eq. 2.2 that are commonly built-in in laser devices [3]. The simplest form of these solutions is associated with a Gaussian-shaped intensity profile, whose peak lies on the optical axis. This is commonly referred to as the fundamental Transverse Electromagnetic Mode (TEM), and is indicated by the designation TEM_{00}. A more general form for the intensity profile can be calculated applying specific boundary conditions. Here we consider the output beam of a laser device with cylindrical symmetric cavity. These beams are described through the combination of a Gaussian function with a generalized Laguerre Polynomial of order p and index l, i.e. L_p^l. Assuming a cylindrical reference frame (r, φ, z), with z denoting the beam axis, r and φ being the polar coordinates in a plane transverse to z, the optical power density is given by [4]:

$$I_{pl}(r, \varphi, z) = I_0 \rho^l \left[L_p^l(\rho)\right]^2 \cos^2(l\varphi) \exp(-\rho) \tag{2.3}$$

where $\rho = 2 \cdot r^2 / w^2(z)$. The quantity $w(z)$ is called the spot size of the Gaussian Beam, defined as the radius at which the intensity of the TEM_{00} mode is $1/e^2$ of its peak value I_0. This set of solutions is commonly referred to as TEM_{lp}. The order and the index of the Laguerre polynomial determine the shape of the intensity profile, as shown in Fig. 2.4.

TEM_{00} beams present several interesting properties. The intensity profile of these beams maintain a Gaussian shape regardless of the selection of the cross section along the propagation axis z. Furthermore, these beams present a relatively low divergence; this is a measure of how large the variation of the spot size $w(z)$ is along z. This concept is illustrated in Fig. 2.5, where the $w(z)$ is plotted. The spot size $w(z)$ of the beam follows an hyperbolic law, and presents a global minimum w_0 where

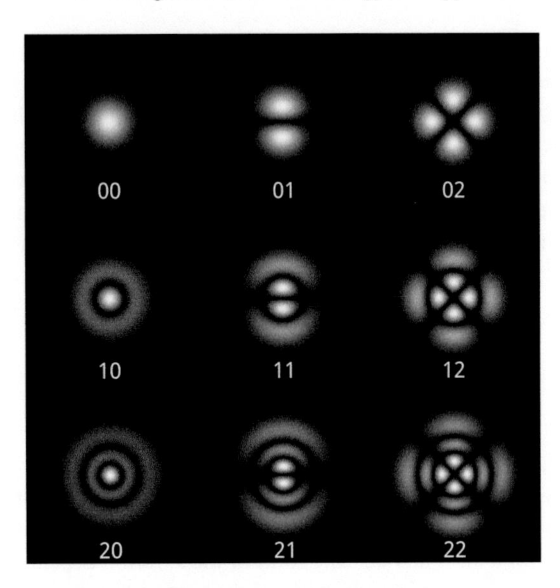

Fig. 2.4 Transverse modes of Gaussian Beams for different values of l and p. Higher values of intensity are represented with brighter shades of *gray*

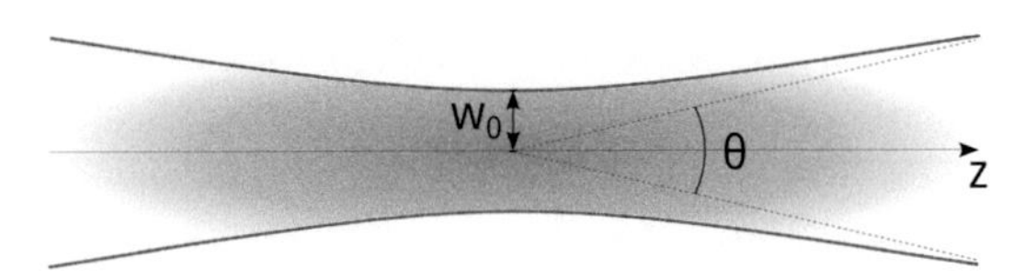

Fig. 2.5 Propagation of a TEM_{00} beam along an optical axis z. The divergence angle θ is shown, which is related to the variation of the spot size of the beam $w(z)$. The spot size measured at the maximum focusing point is denoted with w_0 and is called the beam waist

the focusing reaches its maximum. This quantity is known as the *beam waist*. The divergence angle θ is defined in terms of w_0 and the wavelength λ, i.e.,

$$\theta = \frac{2\lambda}{\pi w_0}. \tag{2.4}$$

From this relation it follows that the divergence increases linearly with the wavelength of the laser beam. Also, the divergence of a beam is inversely proportional to the beam waist w_0. It should be noted that collimated beams of light could be produced also through incoherent light sources. However, this requires the use of a focusing optical system that would greatly attenuate the energy density of the output. In contrast, the collimation of a laser beam does not entail significant losses of optical power, thus permitting the creation of large energy densities even at low output power.

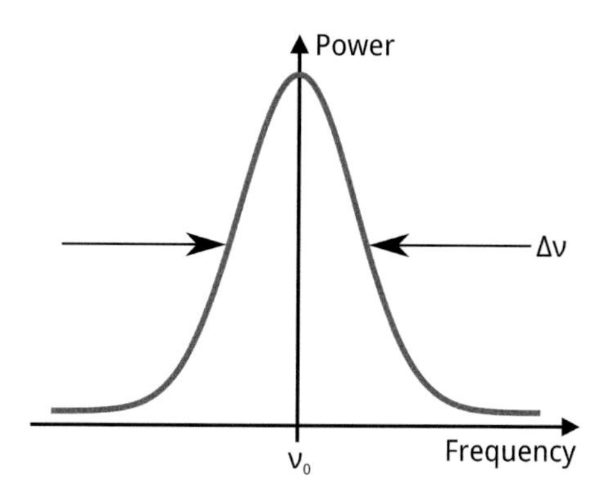

Fig. 2.6 Exemplary laser emission spectrum, centered at ν_0 and with Frequency Spread $\Delta\nu$

2.2.2 *Spectral Properties of Laser Light*

The light generated by a laser device is *coherent*, i.e. the EM waves that form a laser beam bear a fixed phase relationship to each other, thus presenting a high degree of correlation. Laser radiation presents both spatial and temporal coherence. The former refers to the property that the phase difference measured between any pair of points on the wavefront is uniform. Similarly, temporal coherence indicates that the phase of a wave remains constant through time. The coherence of laser light is a direct result of the stimulated emission process, as the emitted photons present the same phase, frequency and direction of stimulating photons [2].

It can be shown that high temporal coherence entails a narrow emission spectrum [2]—this explains why laser devices appear to produce nearly monochromatic light. Typical values of frequency spread $\Delta\nu$ (Fig. 2.6) for a laser range from 1 GHz down to a few Hertz, depending on the properties of the active medium and the design of the cavity. Laser devices are commonly described by the wavelength λ associated with the center ν_0 of their emission spectrum. For instance, most medical carbon dioxide (CO_2) lasers present an emission in the mid-infrared range, centered at 10.6 μm [5].

2.3 Fundamentals of Laser-Matter Interaction

Because of its unique properties, laser radiation interacts with matter differently with respect to the light emitted by a traditional incoherent light source. Laser-matter interaction is an active area of research, which aims to investigate and understand the manifold physical phenomena that occur when matter is exposed to laser light. Most of these phenomena have been extensively studied and reviewed in numerous scholarly works [5–7].

Mechanisms of laser-matter interaction have been classified in various ways in the literature. Here, we start our discussion presenting general concepts related to

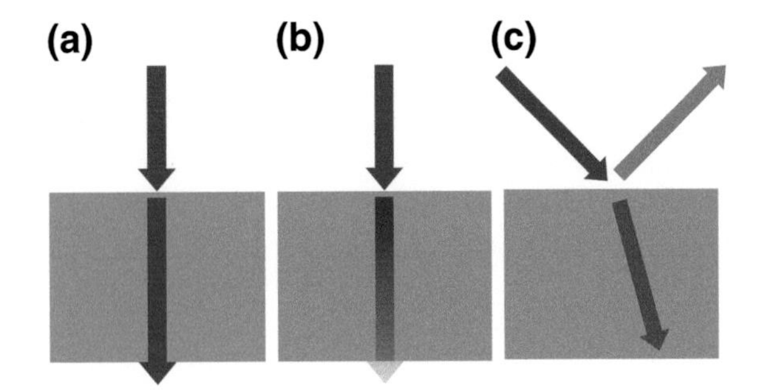

Fig. 2.7 Basic interactions of laser light with matter. Here, the beam is directed onto the surface of a block of material. Depending on the properties of the beam and the material, three different interaction mechanisms may occur: (**a**) Transmission (**b**) Attenuation (**c**) Reflection and Refraction

how matter affects the propagation of a laser beam. When laser light is incident on a material, three basic effects can be observed, as illustrated in Fig. 2.7:

- **Transmission** refers to the undisturbed propagation of light through the material. The material is said to be *transparent*: light travels through it without any attenuation, maintaining the same direction of propagation. The energy density entering the medium equals the one that escapes it.
- **Attenuation** occurs when the energy associated with the laser beam is lost within the material volume. The propagation of the beam through the material results in an attenuation of its energy density, either because energy is absorbed by the material or it is dispersed into it. Basic attenuation mechanisms are *absorption* and *scattering* [5].
- **Reflection and Refraction** occur when light crosses the boundary between materials with different optical properties. A fraction of the incident wave is returned from the surface of the material (reflection), while the remaining part propagates into it (refraction). Refraction is usually associated with a change in the speed and direction of propagation. Reflection and refraction are strongly related to each other by the Fresnel's Equations [8].

In general, these effects might occur simultaneously in a combined fashion, i.e. when light impinges on the surface of a material part of it is reflected, part is transmitted and part is either absorbed or dispersed into the material. The proportions of light which is transmitted, returned or dispersed are dictated by the incident wavelength and the optical properties of the material. The principle of energy conservation holds: the sum of the energies associated with each of these interactions gives the total amount of incident energy.

In the scope of this doctoral thesis, we shall focus on a specific set of laser-matter interactions, in which the target material consists of biological tissue. Most relevant *laser-tissue interactions* are induced by the absorption of laser energy within the tissue volume. Among these, thermal interactions play a crucial role in laser surgery, as we will find later on. In the next section, we present the fundamentals of laser-tissue interaction mechanisms, with particular focus on the effects that laser radiation can produce on tissues.

2.4 Interactions of Lasers with Biological Tissues

Biological tissues are optically *turbid* materials: absorption and scattering dominate the interactions of these media, thus enabling an energy transfer process from the laser source to the tissue [5]. The capability of laser light to penetrate a tissue and deposit energy within its volume is the key of numerous therapeutic applications: lasers can be employed to precisely deliver an energy dose to a selected target volume within an organ, e.g. to destroy malignant tissue. In these applications, the spatial distribution of energy induced by the laser is essential for the purpose of predicting successful treatment. Such distribution is described by the volumetric energy density E_v ($J \cdot m^{-3}$), and depends on the incident wavelength as well as on the optical properties of the target [5, 9].

Relevant optical properties of tissues include the coefficients of absorption μ_a (m^{-1}) and scattering μ_s (m^{-1}). The former determines the fraction of incident energy absorbed by the tissue; the latter is related to how deep laser radiation penetrates into the tissue. Both coefficients are determined by the molecular composition of the target. Because different molecules respond selectively to different wavelengths, these coefficients are wavelength-dependent [10]: for instance, Fig. 2.8 presents the absorption spectra of three different types of human tissues, namely skin, aortic wall and cornea. In the considered range of wavelengths, skin presents the largest absorption due to the presence of melanin molecules, which are known to strongly absorb radiation in the visible range (wavelength: 400–780 nm) [5, 9]. The absorption of aortic tissue is characterized by haemoglobin, which is also a strong absorber in this range. Conversely, cornea does not have any constituent that presents a significant absorbance, thus resulting almost transparent. In general, different types of tissues present different absorption and scattering coefficients. Numerous works

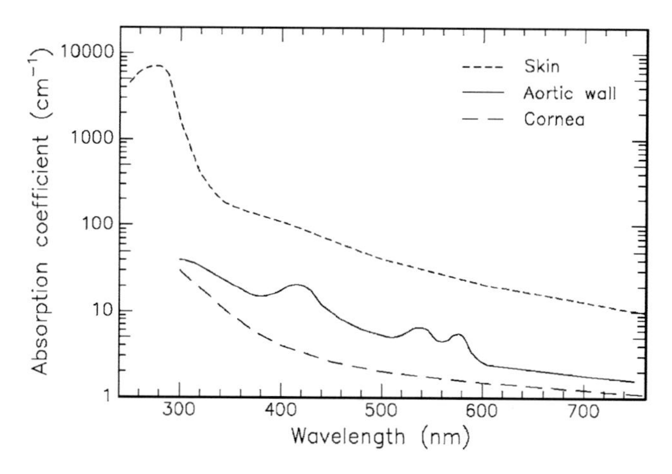

Fig. 2.8 Wavelength-dependency of the absorption coefficients of skin, aortic wall, and cornea. Reproduced from [5] with kind permission from Springer Science+Business Media

report tabulated values of these coefficients sampled on various tissues and for different wavelengths [10]. Nonetheless, slight variations from the reported values may be observed in practice, due to the inherent inhomogeneity of biological tissues: these may present variations in blood content, water content, fiber development, etc. [5, 10].

Laser energy can act on tissues, inducing alterations at the physical and chemical levels. Diverse effects can be produced, depending on the optical properties of tissues discussed above, as well as on the properties that characterize the laser beam: wavelength, beam intensity and waist. Another important parameter is the total time of laser exposure: this is often used in conjunction with the beam intensity to classify laser-tissue interactions, as shown in Fig. 2.9. Five main interaction classes can be distinguished, namely *photodisruption, plasma-induced ablation, photoablation, thermal interactions* and *photochemical interactions* [5]. It is interesting to observe all these interactions occur for similar values of the applied energy density, i.e. between 1 and 1000 J $\cdot$ cm^{-2}. This result shows the practical importance of the exposure time, which can be tuned to selectively enable a specific interaction [5].

For the purpose of this dissertation we shall focus on thermal interactions. For further details on the other types of interactions, the reader is referred to [5].

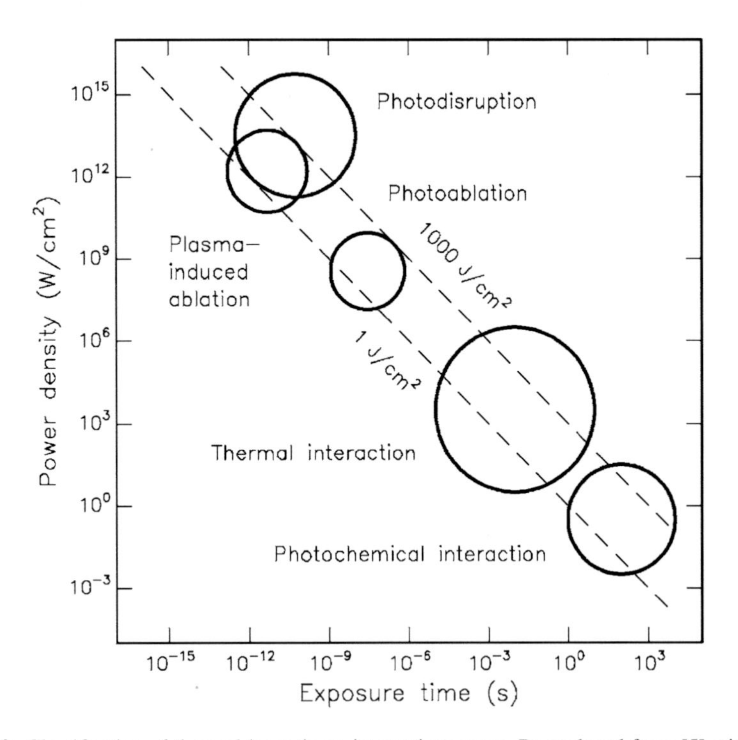

Fig. 2.9 Classification of thermal laser-tissue interactions types. Reproduced from [5] with kind permission from Springer Science+Business Media

2.4.1 Thermal Interactions

Thermal interactions constitute a large group of interaction types, characterized by irradiations longer than 1 μs and shorter than 1 min. During these interactions, laser energy is absorbed by the tissue under the form of heat, thereby determining a local increase of temperature [5]. As we shall see later on, several different effects can be produced on tissue, depending on the duration and peak value of temperature achieved. These effects range from hyperthermia (45 °C) to vaporization (100 °C) and carbonization (>100 °C).

In the scope of laser surgery, laser-induced thermal effects are especially of importance. Vaporization is the process by means of which laser incisions are conducted: because soft tissues are largely composed by water, their molecules start to evaporate at approximately 100 °C, determining a material removal (ablation) process. Although some laser-induced effects are advantageous, others are considered detrimental. It it the case of carbonization, that occurs at temperatures above 100 °C. Carbonization determines the formation of scar tissue, thus diminishing the quality of the surgical procedure. It is important to note that temperature is the parameter that governs the onset of these effects. Therefore, for the purpose of understanding the diverse thermal effects that lasers can produce on tissues, we must establish a model for the spatial and temporal evolution of tissue temperature during laser irradiation. In the following paragraphs we derive the equations that govern the generation of heat within the tissue and see how the generation of heat is related to the variation of temperature. Then, we will review and discuss the diverse thermal effects that lasers can produce on tissues.

Let us consider a sample of homogeneous tissue exposed to a TEM_{00} laser beam, as depicted in Fig. 2.10. For the sake of simplicity, we assume that the surface of tissue exposed to the beam is plain and normally oriented with respect to it. A cylindrical reference frame (r, ϑ, z) is used to describe the tissue geometry, with z being coincident with the beam axis and r representing the radial distance with respect to such axis. Without any loss of generality, cylindrically symmetry is assumed. The

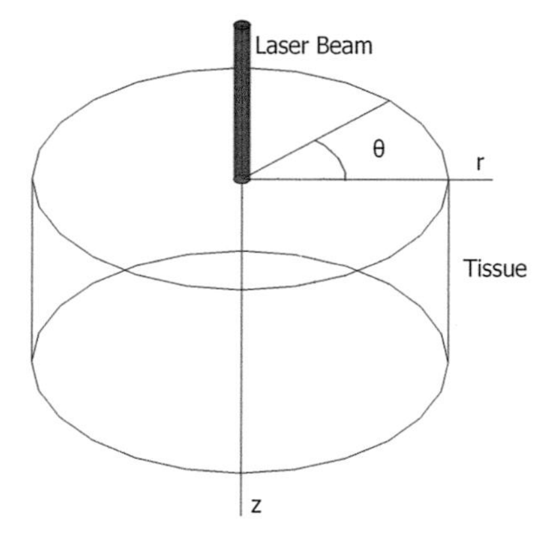

Fig. 2.10 Tissue geometry. Adapted from [11]

beam intensity inside the tissue is then described by Niemz [5]:

$$I(r, z, t) = I_0 \exp\left(-\frac{2r^2}{\omega^2} - \mu_a z\right) \exp\left(\frac{-8t^2}{\tau^2}\right), \tag{2.5}$$

where I_0 is the beam intensity incident on the surface of tissue, μ_a is the coefficient of absorption of the tissue, ω is the beam waist, t is the total exposure time and τ is the pulse duration. This model of intensity does not take into account the effect of scattering, which can be neglected for most practical applications on soft tissues [5]. One important parameter associated with the spatial distribution of intensity within the tissue is the *absorption length*, defined as the inverse of the absorption coefficient μ_a:

$$L = \frac{1}{\mu_a}. \tag{2.6}$$

The absorption length measures the distance, along the beam axis z, at which the intensity has dropped to $1/e$ of its incident value I_0 [5].

The rate of heat generation within the tissue $S(r, z, t)$ ($W \cdot m^{-3}$) is proportional to the intensity I, with the coefficient of absorption μ_a being the proportional factor [5]:

$$S(r, z, t) = \mu_a I(r, z, t). \tag{2.7}$$

Having identified a model for the rate of heat generation, we now focus on the equations that permit to quantify the consequent variation of temperature [5]. Assuming that neither phase transitions (e.g. vaporization) nor tissue alterations (e.g. coagulation) occur, a basic law of thermodynamics can be used to model the change of temperature dT related to a variation of heat content dQ:

$$dT = \frac{dQ}{mc}, \tag{2.8}$$

where m is the mass of tissue, and c is its specific heat capacity, expressed in $J \cdot kg^{-1} \cdot K^{-1}$. A variation of heat content can occur either because of the energy deposited by the heat source (Eq. 2.7) or due to heat conduction, i.e. the variation of heat content per unit of volume ($\dot{q}$), which is the primary mechanism by which heat is transferred to tissue structures not reached by the laser radiation. Other heat losses as heat convection and heat radiation can be neglected in first approximation [5].

It can be shown, by means of the *equation of continuity*[1] and the *general diffusion equation*,[2] that the volumetric variation of heat $\dot{q}$ depends on the temperature by the following relation:

$$\dot{q} = k \Delta T, \tag{2.9}$$

[1]The *equation of continuity* establishes the relation between the heat flow and the temporal change in heat content per unit of volume, $\dot{q}$.

[2]The *general diffusion equation* states that the heat flow is proportional to the temperature gradient.

where Δ is the Laplace operator and k is the *tissue heat conductivity*, expressed in W · m · K. Combining Eq. 2.9 into Eq. 2.8 yields:

$$\dot{T} = \frac{1}{mc}\dot{Q} = \frac{1}{\rho c}\frac{\dot{Q}}{V} = \frac{1}{\rho c}\dot{q} = \frac{1}{\rho c}k\Delta T \tag{2.10}$$

where V is the volume of the tissue (m^3), ρ is the tissue density ($kg \cdot m^{-3}$) and c is its specific heat capacity ($J \cdot kg^{-1}\ K^{-1}$). Equation 2.10 can be extended to account for the heat generated by the laser:

$$\dot{T} = \frac{1}{\rho c}\left(k\Delta T + S\right). \tag{2.11}$$

Using the Laplace operator for the cylindrical reference frame, we obtain:

$$\dot{T} = \kappa\left(\frac{\partial^2}{\partial r^2} + \frac{\partial^2}{r\partial r} + \frac{\partial^2}{\partial z^2}\right)T + \frac{1}{\rho c}S. \tag{2.12}$$

Here, κ is the *temperature conductivity* of tissue, which relates both constants, the specific heat capacity (k) and the heat conductivity (c). Azimuth symmetry is evidenced in the expression above. Exact solution of this inhomogeneous differential equation is rather complex. It involves the use of several approximations and assumptions, as we shall see in greater detail in Chap. 4. Numerical methods are commonly used to solve the time-dependent function that describes the temperature $T(r, z, t)$.

The diffusion of heat within tissue during laser irradiation is described by the *thermal penetration depth* d_{therm} [5]:

$$d_{therm} = \sqrt{4\kappa t}. \tag{2.13}$$

Analogously to the optical absorption length (Eq. 2.6), this term quantifies the depth at which the temperature has dropped to $1/e$ of the superficial value, i.e. with respect to $T(z = 0)$. Equating the optical absorption length with the thermal penetration depth, we obtain the following time-dependent relation:

$$\frac{1}{\mu_a} = \sqrt{4\kappa t}, \tag{2.14}$$

whose solution τ_{therm} is called the *thermal relaxation time*. This quantity gives an indication of how quickly a tissue dissipates the heat generated by a laser. For laser exposures shorter than τ_{therm}, we have that $L > d_{therm}$, i.e. the diffusion of heat is contained in the volume reached by the laser radiation. By contrast, exposure times longer than τ_{therm} determine a significant diffusion of heat also to surrounding tissues, which are not under direct laser irradiation. As we shall see in the following, this result has great practical relevance: it gives a criterion for the selection of the laser exposure time, based on the thermal effects one wants to achieve.

Having established the equations that govern the thermal response of tissues subject to laser irradiation, we now focus on the different biological effects that a thermal interaction may produce. Depending on the duration and peak value of temperature achieved, different effects like coagulation, vaporization, carbonization, and melting may be distinguished. These effects are listed in Table 2.2, together with the temperature at which they occur. Elevating the temperature of tissue up to 60 °C does not induce any permanent alteration, given that this condition is maintained for a time duration in the range of seconds [5]. Above 60 °C [5], coagulation occurs. This is a form of irreversible tissue necrosis which causes cells to cease their function. A phase transition is induced at 100 °C: this is temperature at which the the free water molecules in the tissue start to vaporize. As the volume of water tends to increase during the transition, a pressure build-up occurs. Increasing pressure eventually leads to micro explosions that tear up the fabric of tissue and produce craters. In the literature, this process is commonly referred to as *thermal decomposition* [5]. Another effect that may occur during a thermal interaction is carbonization. This occurs when the tissue temperature rises above 100 °C, i.e. when laser irradiation continues after the water content of tissue has been completely evaporated.

Medical applications of lasers typically aim to induce one specific thermal effect on tissue. Vaporization is exploited in laser surgery to create ablations and produce incisions on tissue [5, 12, 13]. In practice, several thermal effects might occur simultaneously, depending on the parameters that characterize the laser irradiation. The locations and extent of each effect follows the spatial distribution of temperature produced during and after the laser exposure [5]. The coincidence of diverse thermal artifacts is represented in Fig. 2.11, which shows a sample laser incision produced with a CO_2 laser on ex-vivo chicken muscle tissue. The incision line was created through repeated scans of the laser beam: the high temperatures induced in correspondence of the laser incidence points determined the ablation of tissue. Carbonized tissue can be recognized in the surroundings of the incision crater, where the temperature of tissue has risen above 100 °C. These areas appear darker in color with respect to normal tissue. Visual inspection of a broader area around the incision line

Table 2.2 Thermal effects of laser radiation on tissues. Reproduced from [5] with kind permission from Springer Science+Business Media

Temperature (°C)	Biological effect
37	None
45	Hyperthermia
50	Reduction in enzyme activity, cell immobility
60	Denaturation of proteins and collagen, coagulation
80	Permeabilization of membranes
100	Vaporization
>100	Carbonization
>300	Melting

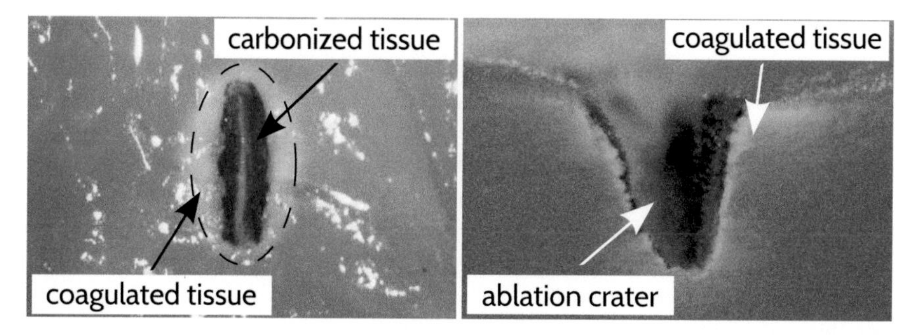

Fig. 2.11 Thermal effects of CO_2 laser radiation on soft tissue. Here, the same tissue specimen is shown from a top view (*left*) and cross-section (*right*) perspective. Material ablation can be observed in correspondence with the laser incision line. Dark areas on the edges of the ablation crater indicate that temperatures over 100 °C have been reached, resulting in the carbonization of tissue. Coagulation can be also be observed, in the surroundings of the laser incision site.The volumetric extent of coagulation has been highlighted in the cross-section image through the use of a fluorescent light source

reveals the presence of coagulated tissue. A temperature below than 100 °C has been induced in these areas by means of heat conduction.

2.4.2 Applications to Clinical Surgery

Lasers are employed in a number of surgical specialties as cutting tools. Their use has gained popularity in those procedures where high accuracy is required, e.g. for the surgical treatment of glottic cancer [13]. With respect to traditional cutting tools, lasers present numerous advantages: they operate in a contact-less fashion, thus ensuring sterile conditions on the surgical site. In surgery of soft tissues, lasers can be tuned to simultaneously cut and coagulate blood, thus preventing excessive blood losses and limiting the need to resort to transfusions; this heamostatic effect further allows to keep the surgical site clean, enhancing the surgeon's assessment of the state of tissues [12, 14, 15]. Furthermore, lasers have enabled the development of new surgical techniques, such as the *piece-wise tumor resection* introduced by Steiner [14], which would have been impossible without a tool able to cut and coagulate surrounding tissues at the same time.

The knowledge of the absorbing and scattering properties of tissues is of paramount importance in laser surgery. Clinicians seek to create clean ablations with minimal thermal damage to surrounding tissues. The selection of a laser source with an appropriate wavelength is an essential prerequisite to achieve these goals. The CO_2 laser is often indicated for surgery of soft tissues. These are rich in water, which is a strong absorber of the infrared radiation emitted by these class of lasers (wavelength: 10.6 μm). Alternatively, the solid-state Er:YAG laser (wavelength: 2940 nm) is recommended for the ablation of bony tissue [5, 16].

For surgical applications of lasers, carbonization of tissues surrounding the ablation site should be minimized as much as possible. It represents a non-intentional damage where healthy tissue that should have been preserved is being compromised, i.e. burned. Carbonization causes a longer recovery time for the patient and may leave scars, diminishing the quality of the procedure [12]. One common strategy to limit the extent of carbonization consists in the selection of laser exposure times shorter than the thermal relaxation time of tissue. In most soft tissues, laser irradiations shorter than 1 μs do not produce significant thermal damage (this simple practical result is referred to as the "1 μs rule") [5]. State-of-the-art CO_2 surgical lasers present minimum pulse durations of a few hundred microseconds [13], thus potentially enabling thermal damage of surrounding tissues.

Laser surgery requires the dexterity to control the laser effects on tissues in order to obtain global appropriate results. These aspects will be discussed in detail in the next chapter. We shall see how the equipment currently in use for laser microsurgeries gives little support to clinicians to detect and understand the effects of laser actions.

References

1. R. Haglund, The properties of light, ed. by F. Träger, in *Springer Handbook of Lasers and Optics* (Springer, New York, 2007), pp. 3–32
2. O. Svelto, S. Longhi, G. Valle, S. Kück, G. Huber, M. Pollnau, H. Hillmer, S. Hansmann, R. Engelbrecht, H. Brand, J. Kaiser, A. Peterson, R. Malz, S. Steinberg, G. Marowsky, U. Brinkmann, D. Lo, A. Borsutzky, H. Wähter, M. Sigrist, E. Saldin, E. Schneidmiller, M. Yurkov, K. Midorikawa, J. Hein, R. Sauerbrey, and J. Helmcke, Lasers and coherent light sources, ed. by F. Träger, in *Springer Handbook of Lasers and Optics* (Springer, New York, 2007), pp. 583–936
3. N. Lindlein, G. Leuchs, Wave optics, ed. by F. Trägerin, in *Springer Handbook of Lasers and Optics* (Springer, New York, 2007), pp. 87–156
4. W. Koechner, Optical resonator, in *Solid-State Laser Engineering*. Springer Series in Optical Sciences, vol. 1 (Springer New York, 2006), pp. 210–299
5. M. Niemz, *Laser-tissue Interactions* (Springer, Berlin, 2004)
6. M. Allmen, *Laser-Beam Interactions with Materials: Physical Principles and Applications*, Springer Series in Materials Science (Springer, Berlin, 2012)
7. D. Bäuerle, *Laser Processing and Chemistry* (Springer, Berlin, 2011)

8. M. Brinkmann, J. Hayden, M. Letz, S. Reichel, C. Click, W. Mannstadt, B. Schreder, S. Wolff, S. Ritter, M. Davis, T. Bauer, H. Ren, Y.-H. Fan, S.-T. Wu, K. Bonrad, E. Krätzig, K. Buse, R. Paquin, Optical materials and their properties, ed. by F. Träger, in *Springer Handbook of Lasers and Optics* (Springer, New York, 2007), pp. 249–372
9. A. Vogel, V. Venugopalan, Mechanisms of pulsed laser ablation of biological tissues. Chem. Rev. **103**(2), 577–644 (2003)
10. S.L. Jacques, Optical properties of biological tissues: a review. Phys. Med. Biol. **58**(11), R37 (2013)
11. L. Fichera, D. Pardo, L. Mattos, Modeling tissue temperature dynamics during laser exposure, ed. by I. Rojas, G. Joya, J. Cabestany, in *Advances in Computational Intelligence*. Lecture Notes in Computer Science, vol. 7903 (Springer, Berlin, 2013), pp. 96–106. http://dx.doi.org/10.1007/978-3-642-38682-4_12 (Online)
12. R. Steiner, Laser-tissue interactions, in *Laser and IPL Technology in Dermatology and Aesthetic Medicine*, ed. by C. Raulin, S. Karsai (Springer, Berlin, 2011), pp. 23–36
13. M. Rubinstein, W. Armstrong, Transoral laser microsurgery for laryngeal cancer: a primer and review of laser dosimetry. Lasers Med. Sci. **26**(1), 113–124 (2011)
14. W. Steiner, P. Ambrosch, Endoscopic laser surgery of the upper aerodigestive tract: with special emphasis on cancer surgery. Thieme (2000)
15. V. Oswal, M. Remacle, Transoral laser laryngeal surgery, in *Principles and Practice of Lasers in Otorhinolaryngology and Head and Neck*, 2nd edn., ed. by O. Vasant, R. Marc (Kugler Publications, Amsterdam, The Netherlands, 2014), pp. 99–116
16. C. Apel, R. Franzen, J. Meister, H. Sarrafzadegan, S. Thelen, N. Gutknecht, Influence of the pulse duration of an er: yag laser system on the ablation threshold of dental enamel. Lasers Med. Sci. **17**(4), 253–257 (2002)

Chapter 3
Cognitive Supervision for Transoral Laser Microsurgery

The thermal laser-tissue interactions described in Chap. 2 constitute the basic building block of laser microsurgery. In particular, ablation by vaporization is the process by means of which laser incisions and resections are performed. As we shall see in this chapter, these interactions need to be carefully monitored to ensure the formation of incisions as planned by the surgeon. Control of the laser effects on tissue is essential for the purpose of ensuring a safe and efficient surgical performance, which encompasses both resection accuracy and limited thermal damage to underlying and surrounding tissues.

Despite its importance, the control of the laser effects on tissues during Transoral Laser Microsurgery (TLM) is still performed manually, since available technologies do not include any support to monitor the state of tissues under laser irradiation. When analyzing the workflow of these interventions, it becomes apparent that the quality of laser resections depends entirely on clinicians, who must possess the experience required to anticipate and understand the results of their laser actions.

This chapter introduces the problem of the automatic supervision of laser-induced effects during laser surgery. A top-down approach is used to tackle this problem: specific circumstances in which surgeons would value enhanced information regarding the effects of their laser actions on tissues are identified. The problem is grounded in the identification of variables of interest that are selected as target for the supervision. In the scope of this thesis, we explore the application of artificial cognitive approaches to monitor these variables in a surgical scenario.

The first two sections of this chapter describe the current workflow of TLM and discuss its limitations from a clinical perspective. Our analysis is based both on evidence reported in medical literature, as well as on the opinions of clinicians who were consulted in the course of this doctoral research. In Sect. 3.3, we formulate the concept of a system capable of assisting clinicians during TLM, enhancing their perception of laser-induced effects on tissues. Two specific effects: thermal (temperature of tissues) and mechanical (laser cutting depth). We will review existing approaches to monitor these effects during laser irradiation, focusing on considerations regarding their

L. Fichera, *Cognitive Supervision for Robot-Assisted Minimally Invasive Laser Surgery*, Springer Theses, DOI 10.1007/978-3-319-30330-7_3

applicability in a TLM setup. To overcome the limitations of existing approaches, we will focus our attention on alternatives based on artificial cognitive methods. Section 3.4 describes our approach, which consists in the application of statistical learning to create models capable of predicting the aforementioned laser effects on tissues. This will lead us to the formulation of the research questions (in Sect. 3.5) that constitute the core of this doctoral dissertation, and that will be addressed in Chaps. 4 and 5. Finally, Sect. 3.6 presents the materials and methods used in our investigation.

3.1 Workflow of Transoral Laser Microsurgery

The typical surgical setup for TLM is represented in Fig. 3.1. The patient is positioned supine on the surgical bed and administered general anesthesia. A laryngoscope is inserted into his oral cavity down to the larynx: this tool consists of a rigid hollow shaft which provides a direct line-of-sight view of the surgical site. Because of the narrow size of the laryngeal lumen, these operations necessitate the use of a microscope: the average width of the larynx is well below 5.0 cm both in adult males and females [1].

The procedure begins with a visual preoperative inspection, aimed to (i) determine the location and extent of the lesion to be excised, and (ii) plan the intervention accordingly. In the example shown in Fig. 3.2a an inspection of the vocal folds is carried out, which reveals the presence of a superficial glottic tumor. To perform a closer analysis of the lesion, the surgeon might alternatively use a camera-equipped endoscopic device, which is delivered through the laryngoscope in proximity of

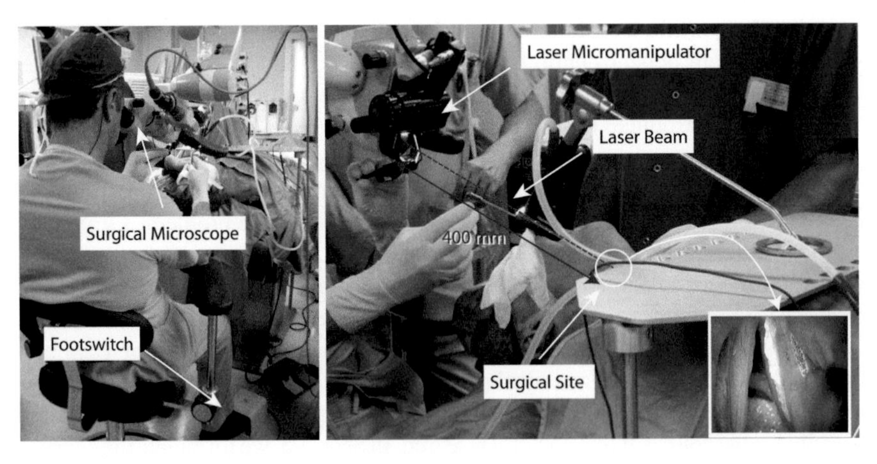

Fig. 3.1 Surgical setup for transoral laser microsurgery. Because of the minuscule size of the operating field, the intervention necessitates the use of a microscope. The laser activation is controlled by the surgeon through a footswitch. In the enlargement on the right, the laser micromanipulator is shown, which allows the surgeon to control the position of the surgical area. Distance between the micromanipulator and the surgical field is 400 mm (normal operating distance). Adapted from [2]

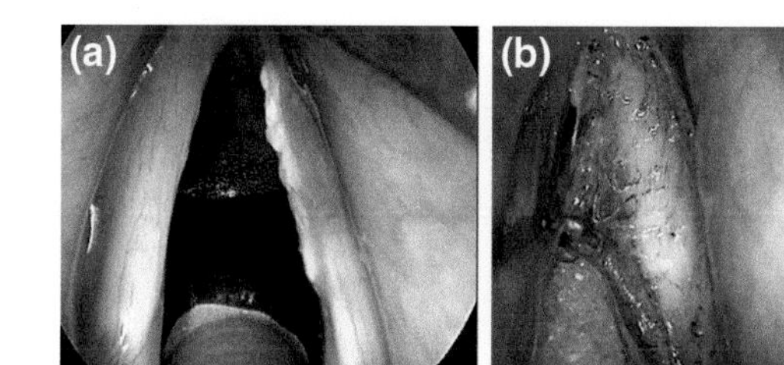

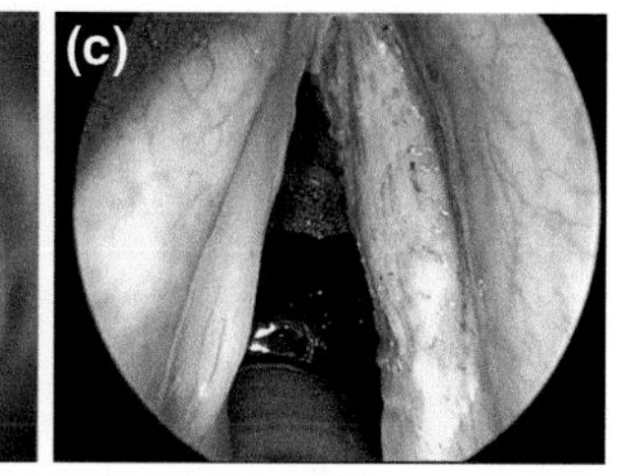

Fig. 3.2 Surgical excision of glottic squamous cell carcinoma. Here the surgical site is visualized through a microscope. The tumor is inspected during a preoperative examination (**a**) it appears as an irregular *white* mass on the surface of the right vocal fold. Tumor resection is shown in (**b**). Forceps are used to apply traction on the tissue, thus exposing the desired resection plane. The final result is shown in (**c**). Images courtesy of Prof. Giorgio Peretti, MD, Clinica Otorinolaringoiatrica, University of Genova

the lesion. During the inspection, the surgeon builds a plan of the procedure to be performed, which entails the selection of an appropriate resection technique and a preliminary mental plan of the dissection.

After the extent of resection has been determined, the tumor is excised with the laser. The carbon dioxide (CO_2) laser (wavelength 10.6 μm) is commonly used in TLM interventions, because of its optimal absorption properties in soft tissues of the larynx [3, 4]. The use of potassium titanyl phosphate (KTP) solid-state lasers (wavelength 532 nm) is also reported in the literature; other types of lasers (thulium, gold) are currently being evaluated [3].

In most surgical equipment, incisions are controlled manually moving the laser beam by means of a mechanical joystick and activating it through a footswitch (see Fig. 3.1) [3]. Forceps are used to apply traction on the tissue, exposing the desired resection plane (as shown in Fig. 3.2b). State-of-the-art laser systems incorporate robotic technology to offer the automatic execution of pre-programmed laser scan patterns. This concept is illustrated in Fig. 3.3: the coordination of one (or more) motorized reflective elements allows to realize diverse scan patterns. Tissue incision by laser scanning has been shown to be superior in terms of quality and accuracy with respect to manual control: laser scanning prevents the accumulation of heat by multi-pass irradiation, thus reducing the risk of thermal damage [6]. Nonetheless, the scanning mirrors commercially available still retain a manual element, i.e. they rely on the use of the traditional joystick to position the scan pattern on the desired incision line [2].

Small, well-delimited tumors are resected en bloc, as it is the case shown in Fig. 3.2b. A different technique is used for larger tumors: these are transected and removed in pieces [4]. It is important to point out that the primary objective of tumor resection is its complete eradication. This is known as *surgical radicality* and is a time-honored principle of surgery, based on the fact that an incomplete resection results in a recurrence of the disease [4]. To achieve sufficient radicality, the tumor is resected with an additional layer of healthy tissue that abuts it. The extent of this layer is decided by the surgeon based on the indications provided by the medical

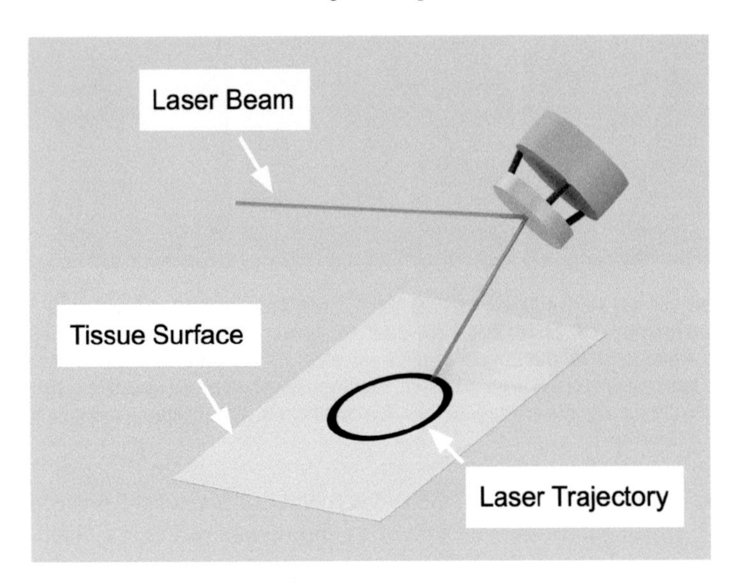

Fig. 3.3 Robotic laser micromanipulation system. The beam is deflected on the target by a 2-DOF steering mirror, which can be controlled to produce automatic laser trajectories. Adapted from [5]

literature: a typical resection margin for Squamous Cell Carcinoma (SCC) of the larynx is at least 5 mm [7, 8]. Once the tumor has been removed, an histological analysis is carried out to verify the appropriateness of the selected resection margins. The outcome of this examination is used to assess the possibility that residual cancer might have been left in situ. If the analysis reports any evidence of cancer in the margins, the physician might decide to repeat the surgical intervention.

Although TLM is primarily concerned with surgical radicality, in practice clinicians attempt to limit the size of the resection margins, in order to preserve as much healthy tissue as possible. This strategy is determined by the application of a second important medical principle, called *function preservation* [4], whose objective is to preserve the functionality of the organs being operated. In order to enable function preservation, the largest possible amount of healthy tissue that is not affected by the tumor should be spared. An example is shown in Fig. 3.2c: the SCC initially diagnosed on the right vocal fold (see Fig. 3.2a) has been resected without compromising the anatomical structure of the vocal fold, thereby allowing the patient to speak normally again after the intervention. Early stage tumors as the one shown in this example are particularly amenable to the application of function preservation strategies, however these may not be applicable in every case. Obtaining cancer-free (clear) margins remains of paramount importance to the aim of the procedure: incremental layers of tissue are removed until an appropriate margin is found [4].

In general, attaining resection margins that fulfill the requirements of both surgical radicality and organ preservation necessitates a correct surgical technique. As we shall see in the next section, this is particularly demanding in TLM.

3.2 Technical Limitations of Transoral Laser Microsurgery

Evidence of clear margins is required for a successful tumor resection, however the margins may be compromised by an inadequate laser cutting technique: lasers induce thermal artifacts on tissue, in the areas that surround the beam incidence point. These effects may be desirable to some extent—for instance, coagulation allows to avoid significant blood losses. Nonetheless, the creation of vast thermal damage might hinder the physician's interpretation of the adequacy of the resection margins both during the operation and the successive histological analysis, undermining any possible assessment of surgical radicality [9]. In this respect, another potential limiting factor is the usage of older surgical laser sources: the evolution of laser technology has led to the construction of ultra-pulsed CO_2 lasers which present narrower bands of thermal damage [6].

When function preservation is the aim, incision accuracy also becomes of fundamental importance. This is the case, for instance, of the resection of glottic tumours, in which reduced resection margins are selected for functional purposes. Typical values for these range between 1 and 2 mm, as larger values would result in a significant damage to the vocal function [7, 8]. To achieve such level of resection accuracy, both the width and depth of laser cuts need to be precisely controlled: to this aim, it is desirable to produce narrow incision widths, while the cutting depth should be as close as possible to the planned one. Even a few millimetres of additional resected tissue would greatly impact the functional outcomes of surgery [4].

The issues introduced above have been discussed with the clinicians involved in this research, during a series of interviews conducted in the initial stages of the μRALP project. From these interviews, it emerged that technologies currently in use for TLM do not include any functionality to support a correct laser cutting technique. As a result, nowadays the quality of resections relies entirely on the dexterity and experience of the clinician. Extensive training is required to develop an effective laser cutting. This includes the acquisition of a basic knowledge of the physical principles behind laser ablation of tissue, and the ability to manipulate the laser dosimetry parameters and its exposure time in order to obtain adequate cutting [3, 4]. Laser parameters used in clinical practice include power, energy delivery mode, pulse duration, incision scanning frequency and exposure time. At present times, no standard recipe exists to determine the parameters and the exposure required to obtain an optimal incision. Physicians use different settings, depending on their skills, experience and preferred technique [3].

Because of its contactless nature, laser surgery represents a challenge to clinicians: the lack of haptic feedback during laser cutting impairs the surgeon's perception of the incision depth and width. Furthermore, the thermal processes that occur during laser ablation are difficult to perceive, potentially leading to undesired tissue damage. Although experienced clinicians normally have sufficient knowledge and understanding of the laser ablation processes, the lack of perception of the effects of lasers on tissues represents a practical problem for many others.

In one of the interviews, we administered a questionnaire[1] aimed at understanding what new technological development clinicians would find most useful in the course of surgery. In their answers, clinicians indicated that technologies capable of monitoring the state of tissues during laser cutting would be useful to overcome the perception issues mentioned above; furthermore, they showed interest in the addition of novel safety functionalities to current laser systems: for instance, having an intelligent laser source that takes over the control of the intensity in selected dangerous circumstances, e.g. when the probability of thermal damage of tissues is high.

3.3 Supervision of the Laser Incision Process

From the evidence presented in the previous section, it emerges that clinicians do not have any technological support to monitor or control the quality of their laser incisions. Of particular interest are (i) thermal laser effects that could ultimately damage the tissues and (ii) the extent of laser resections. Here, we propose the creation of a *supervisory system*, in charge of monitoring these two important processes. The aim of such a system is to complement and enhance the surgeon's perception, providing information that would be difficult or impossible to obtain by visual inspection alone. We expect this will improve the surgeon's control of his laser actions, facilitating the creation of uniform and well-defined incisions, while minimizing thermal damage to surrounding tissues.

The concept of the supervisory system was originally formulated in [10]. The system is divided into two independent modules, each focusing on the monitoring of one of the processes mentioned above. In the following, we shall introduce these modules and discuss the challenges associated with their realization.

3.3.1 Monitoring of Tissue Overheating

This module monitors the temperature of tissues under direct laser irradiation and their surroundings. Figure 3.4 shows the type of supervision this technology may provide. For instance, the surgeon may be provided with an estimation of the temperature of tissues during laser cutting; or, with overheating alerts. Clinicians may use this information, e.g. stopping the cutting process if certain areas of tissue reach excessively high temperatures, and thus are likely to be get necrotic.

Traditional approaches to monitor the temperature of tissue during medical treatments require the placement of sensing equipment in direct contact with the measurement site [11]. These approaches are not applicable during TLM, due to space constraints: the surgical site is accessed through a transoral access which does not offer enough volume for the introduction of additional sensing equipment.

[1]available in Appendix A.

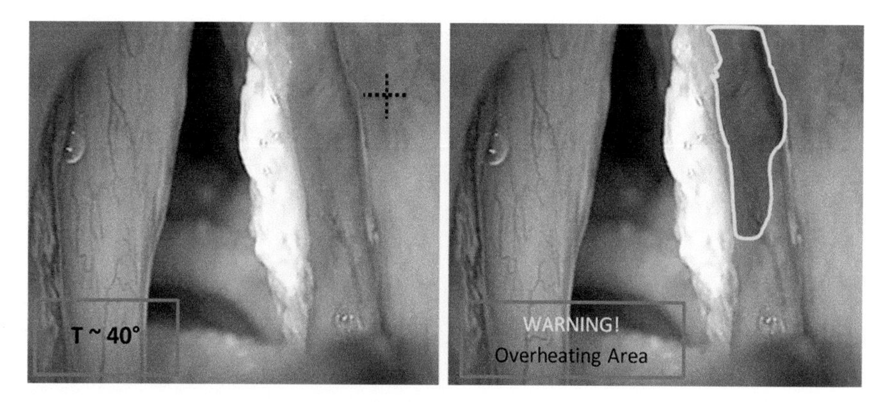

Fig. 3.4 Mock-up showing the on-line monitoring of tissue temperature. This module continuously estimates the superficial temperature of tissues on the surgical site. A cursor can be used to select a point-of-interest, whose temperature should be displayed (*left figure*). Alternatively, the temperature information can be used to issue safety alerts, e.g. if the probability of thermal damage of a zone exceeds a threshold level (*right figure*)

Non-invasive techniques based on common medical imaging technologies are currently being investigated [11]. These may require the introduction of substantial changes to the medical protocol, e.g. the use of MRI-compatible equipment. Furthermore, whether these methods account for the dynamic changes in temperature observed in a spatially concentrated area during laser microsurgery is to be verified.

The dynamics of tissue temperature describes how temperature spreads out in space during laser exposure as times goes on. As we have seen in the previous chapter, this phenomenon is described by the heat diffusion Eq. (2.12). Solutions to this inhomogeneous differential equation depend on the specific form of the input, as well as on the initial and the boundary conditions [12]. Solutions are commonly evaluated by means of numerical methods, as in [13–16]. These studies present models able to predict the temperature of tissue under specific conditions: laser wavelength, tissue type, temperature range. They coincide in saying that the variation of tissue temperature during laser irradiation is a complex phenomenon that involves non-linearities. These types of models are not straightforward to scale into an online predictive technology providing a temperature value of the tissue surface depending on the actions of the surgeon. Furthermore, a considerable number of parameters representing tissue and laser properties must be accounted for when modeling it. Accurate and real-time measurement of some of these parameters is not straightforward in a surgical setup. Laser motion during an incision includes an additional important challenge to the objective of modeling the thermal effects. To the best of our knowledge, none of the available models of temperature dynamics takes into account a scenario with a moving beam.

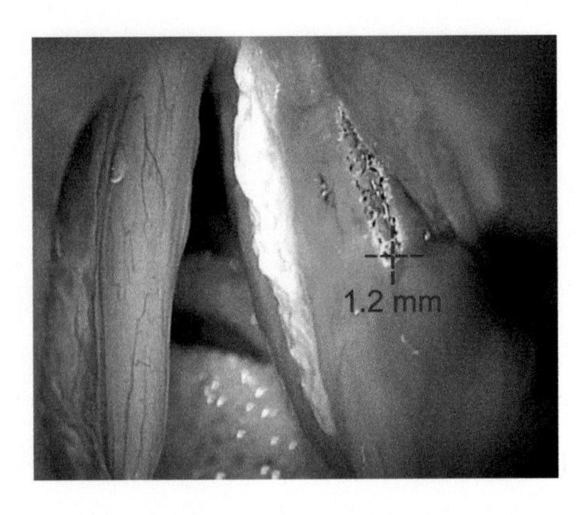

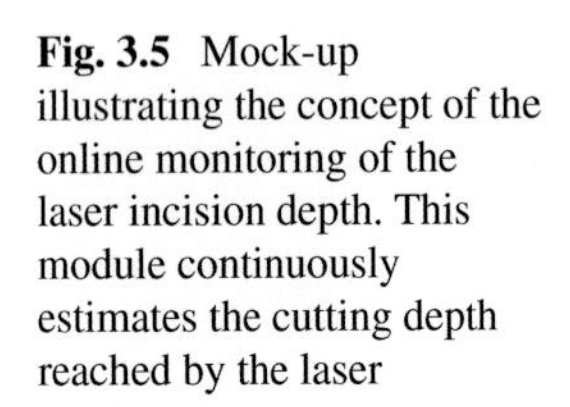
Fig. 3.5 Mock-up illustrating the concept of the online monitoring of the laser incision depth. This module continuously estimates the cutting depth reached by the laser

3.3.2 Monitoring of the Laser Incision Depth

This module monitors the incision depth as it develops during laser cutting. This information could be shown to clinicians (for example, as illustrated in Fig. 3.5), to enhance their perception of the laser cutting process.

Different approaches have been proposed to estimate the amount of tissue removed during laser ablation. However, none of them fulfill the necessary requirements to offer on-line estimation of incision depth. Methods based on mathematical modeling [17] and numerical simulations [18] have provided a viable solution to predict the ablation volume in hard tissue. These methods assume a specific tissue composition and their applicability to soft tissues is yet to be verified. Furthermore, these are computationally intensive and thus not suitable for on-line applications.

Alternative solutions, based on sensing, have been recently developed [19, 20]. Such solutions provide the capability of tracking the ablation crater during laser irradiation, without any *a priori* knowledge on the physical properties of tissue. However these approaches requires the use of additional sensing devices in the proximity of the ablation zone, limiting their applicability in TLM due to space constraints. The small size of the larynx does not offer enough volume for the introduction of additional equipment.

Recent advances in vision-based tissue surface reconstruction [21] seem a promising option to estimate the depth of laser ablation craters intraoperatively.

3.4 Cognitive Models

We propose to investigate the problem of monitoring the state of tissues during laser cutting using a virtual sensing approach [10]; i.e. we theorize that appropriate mathematical models can be used to map the application of laser energy to the resulting effects on tissue (incision depth and temperature variation). The input space of these models coincide with the set of high-level laser inputs used by surgeons to control the laser incision process. The resulting effects on tissue depend on the combination of these parameters plus the total time of laser exposure.

These models are inspired and motivated by the capacity of humans beings to map and fuse diverse sets of information and infer the future state of events. Experienced surgeons possess the skills required to achieve precise and clean laser cutting, yet they certainly do not solve the complex differential equations that govern thermal laser-tissue interactions. This seems to indicate that they have a mental, probably not explicit, estimation about the state of the tissue, on the basis of which they tune the laser parameters and decide the amount of time the tissue should be exposed to the laser. Our intent is to create models that capture and reproduce this skill, mapping the high-level laser inputs to the resulting temperature of tissue and depth of laser incision. The problem of defining models capable of such behavior can be seen as the design of an artificial cognitive model [22].

Cognitive model generally denotes the combination of a knowledge set with a given cognitive architecture [23]. The knowledge captures the experience about a certain process or entity, while the cognitive architecture specifies how this knowledge is represented, acquired, and processed in order to implement some cognitive behavior. In the case of our models, we propose to acquire the necessary knowledge through supervised machine learning techniques.

Machine learning provides the means to approximate the behavior of a system or process without explicitly programming it: such behaviors are instead extracted from sample data. In the framework of statistical learning, knowledge about a process is represented in terms of a *hypothesis function* that describes its input/output characteristic [24]. *Learning* denotes the process of determining the form of the hypothesis function that better describes the process of interest. In a supervised learning setting, this search is performed on the basis of sample input/output pairs, collected during repeated observations of the process. In the next section, we shall formalize two hypothesis functions, aimed to describe laser effects (overheating and incision depth) on tissues during laser cutting. The remainder of the chapter will be dedicated to the materials and methods employed for the collection of the data sets required in the learning task.

3.5 Problem Formulation

Different parameters of the laser source can be manipulated to control the laser incision process. These include laser power (P) and scanning frequency (ω_s). In addition, the laser light can be delivered either as continuous wave or through intermittent pulses, with τ designating the duration of a single light pulse. Here, we model the influence of these parameters and that of the exposure time (t_{exp}) on (i) the superficial temperature of tissue and (ii) the laser incision depth. Our investigation starts out from two hypothesis functions, that are defined in the following subsections. Both hypotheses refer to a simple scenario, involving the laser incision of a slab of tissue.

For the sake of simplicity, we shall assume that the surface S of tissue is flat and smooth, i.e. it presents no irregularities, and that the laser beam is normally incident on it. Furthermore, we will assume that the laser beam is perfectly focused on the tissue surface, i.e. the radius of the laser spot on the surface of tissue equals the beam waist.

3.5.1 Temperature Hypothesis

To obtain an hypothesis that models the temperature dynamics of tissue, we start from a discretization of the surface of tissue into $n \times m$ squared superficial elements.

Definition 3.1 Let us define $\mathbf{T} \in \mathbb{R}^{n \times m}$ as the temperature of a set of $n \times m$ superficial elements.

Hypothesis 1 There exists a function, f, such that

$$\mathbf{T} = f(P, \tau, \omega_s, t_{exp}, \mathbf{T}_0) \quad (3.1)$$

Here, $\mathbf{T}_0$ is the temperature of tissue at the beginning of laser irradiation. Equation 3.1 estimates the temperature at any given point $p \in S$, given the laser parameters and inputs. Learning function f requires a dataset of L samples of the input/output variables $\left\{\mathbf{T}^i, (P, \tau, \omega_s, t_{exp}, \mathbf{T}_0)^i\right\}_{i=1}^{L}$. Based on these, Eq. 3.1 can be approximated using a supervised learning method.

3.5.2 Laser Incision Depth Hypothesis

We now formulate a similar hypothesis for the laser incision depth.

Definition 3.2 Let us define d as the incision depth produced by means of a laser in soft tissue; d identifies the altitude difference between the bottom of the laser crater and the surface of tissue.

Here, we further assume that the depth of incision created by means of laser scans is uniform across the incision width.

Hypothesis 2 There exists a function, f, such that

$$d = f(P, \tau, \omega_s, t_{exp}) \quad (3.2)$$

The model estimates the depth of laser incision based on the used laser parameters and inputs. To learn function f, a dataset $\left\{d^i, (P, \tau, \omega_s, t_{exp})^i\right\}_{i=1}^{L}$ is required.

3.6 Materials and Methods

The datasets required to learn the hypothesis functions (Eqs. 3.1 and 3.2) were collected through a series of controlled experiments. The experimental setup comprises a surgical laser source, which was used to study the effects of the laser parameters on the resulting incision depth and superficial temperature, and to derive the model intended to be used for estimation.

Laser motion and activation were controlled with a computerized system and the resulted incisions were examined under a microscope to measure their depth. Two forms of target: gelatin phantom tissue and ex-vivo chicken muscular tissue were used in the scope of this thesis. Measurement protocols were implemented to obtain the input-output pairs required to derive the forward model based on statistical regression techniques.

3.6.1 Controlled Incision of Soft Tissue

Incisions are produced by moving the laser beam along desired cutting paths on the tissue. Laser scanning, as described in [25], was used for this work: motorized mirrors are used to deflect the laser beam, enabling the automatic execution of pre-programmed cutting patterns. High-frequency cycles of the laser motion across the target tissue remove overlying layers with each pass.

The experimental setup (Fig. 3.6) uses a commercial surgical laser source, the Zeiss Opmilas CO2 25 (wavelength 10.6 μm, TEM_{00} beam profile), whose power is configurable in the range 2 to 25W. In the system used in this research, maximum power density is obtained when the laser spot is focused with a radius of 250 μm. Two energy delivery modes are provided, Continuous Wave (CW) and Repeated Pulse (RP), with the following pulse durations (τ): 0.05s, 0.1s, 0.2s, 0.5s. The concept of energy delivery mode will be further described in the next section. The CW/long-pulsed laser source used in this study has been superseded in clinical practice by short-pulsed (millisecond) lasers, which are known to produce more efficient cutting and reduced thermal damage [3]. However, the use of this equipment does not limit the applicability of the estimation methodology we propose. Our method, in fact, relies on a forward model mapping the laser inputs to the resulting effects on tissue. Thus, it can be applied to any laser source, provided that an appropriate forward model is used.

A motorized micromanipulator system previously developed in our laboratory [25] provides the controlled motion of the laser. This device regulates the motion of the laser through a tip/tilt fast steering mirror (S-334 manufactured by PI GmbH, Germany), with a maximum accuracy of 4 μm at a distance of 400 mm from the target (typical operating distance). The laser source and the micromanipulator are both connected to a Digital Operation Module (E-517 PI GmbH, Germany) which controls the motion and the activation of the laser. A user interface running on a GNU/Linux workstation allows the user to select exposure time, incision length and scanning speed.

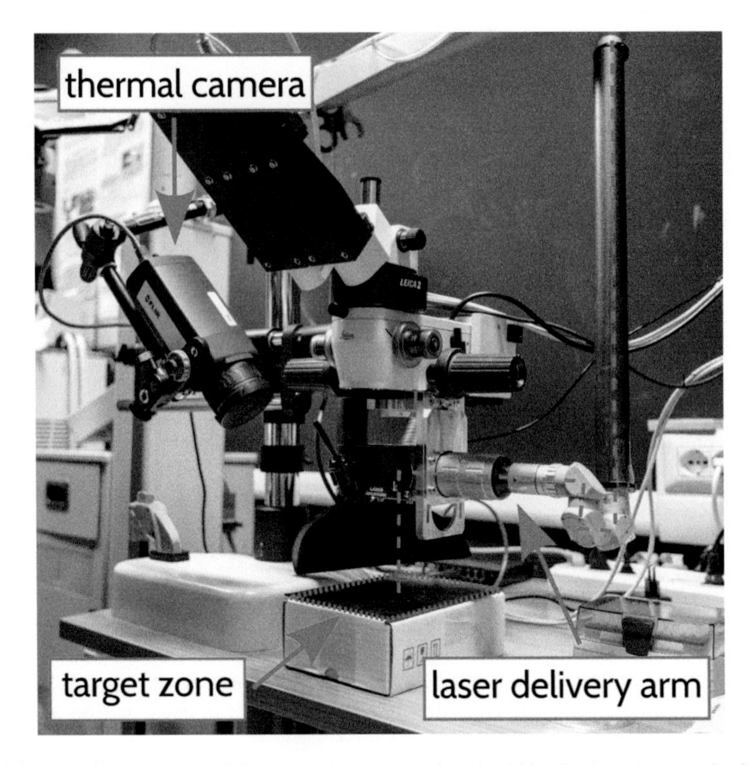

Fig. 3.6 Experimental setup. Tissue specimens are placed within the target zone. An infrared thermal camera (FLIR A655c) is used to monitor the temperature of tissue targets. The laser beam is delivered on the target through a passive articulated arm. A motorized micromanipulator provides the means to control the laser motion. Reproduced from [26] with kind permission from Springer Science+Business Media

3.6.2 Tissue Targets

Initial incision trials were conducted on tissue phantoms. Cylindrical agar-based gel targets were produced to mimic soft tissue. The constituents used to fabricate these targets are deionized water and agar powder (B&V s.r.l., Italy). The concentrations are as follows: 98 % water, 2 % agar. In soft tissues, the absorption of infrared laser radiation is dominated by the presence of free water molecules [12], therefore water was chosen as the main constituent of the targets. Although different from tissue, these gels offer a controlled medium on which the effects of the laser can be reproducibly studied [27].

In order to gather the data required for the learning tasks, additional incision trials were performed on fresh ex-vivo chicken muscle tissue. Like most soft tissues, chicken breast has a high water content, which makes it a convenient target for CO_2 laser ablation trials. Before the experiments, tissue samples were kept for 20 min in an open refrigerated box at a controlled temperature (7–12 °C), in order to preserve their moisture and prevent degradation. To ensure identical initial temperature, the samples were monitored with an infrared thermal camera (Fig. 3.6). It is important to point out that the ex-vivo model selected in this study does not present the same laser absorption of in-vivo tissues. The thermal effects of a laser on living tissues is influenced by several factors that are not present in ex-vivo models [12], e.g. heat convection due to blood perfusion. Nonetheless, most of these factors can be neglected in first approximation [12]. The selection of an ex-vivo model is consistent with the objective of this study, i.e. to prove the concept of an on-line depth estimation system based on statistical regression analysis.

3.6.3 Measurement of Temperature During Laser Irradiation

Temperature of the surface of tissue is captured continuously during laser exposure plus a proportional time after the laser is turning off in order to capture the cooling down process. A digital thermal camera (FLIR A655, Flir Systems Inc., USA) equipped with a filter for CO_2 emissions. Data collected from the sensor is a stream of video frames with a resolution of 640×480 pixels at a rate of 100 Hz. A sample frame is shown in Fig. 3.7. The distance from the camera to the tissue was maintained constant throughout the experiments. At this distance, each pixel covers an area of $0.177 \times 0.177\,\text{mm}^2$.

3.6.4 Measurement of Depth of Incision

To examine the ablation craters, we used a digital microscope (Olympus SZX16). In order to get a complete exposure of the crater profile, tissue targets were sectioned into slices. Agar-based targets were sectioned manually with a blade. Ex-vivo soft

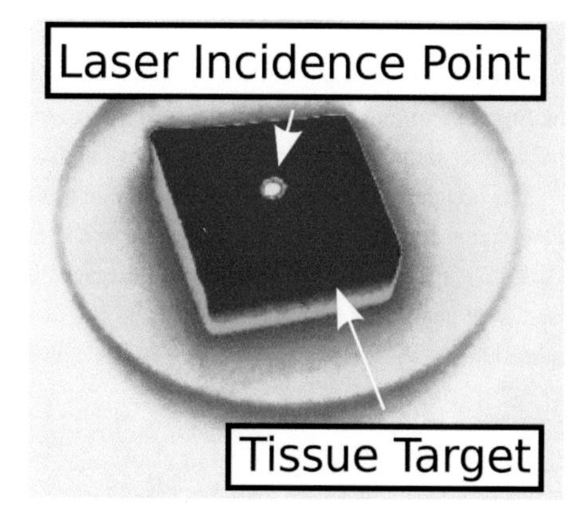

Fig. 3.7 Raw thermal image of phantom tissue target during laser irradiation. Brighter colors represent higher values of temperature. Reproduced from [26] with kind permission from Springer Science+Business Media

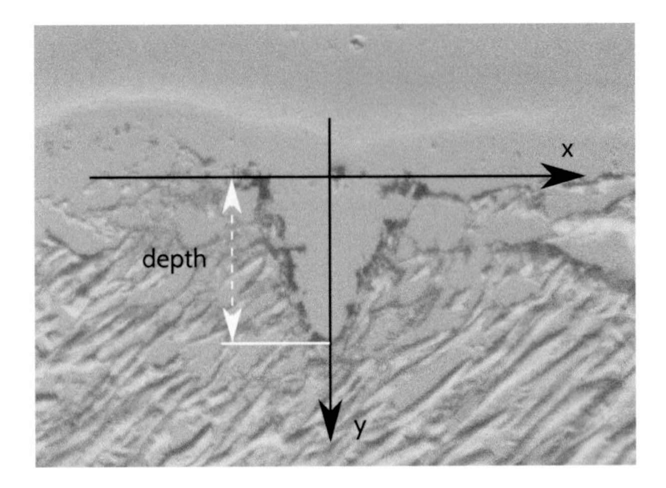

Fig. 3.8 Frozen section of chicken muscle tissue after laser ablation. The frame used for the measurement of the ablation depth is shown. Reproduced from [28] with kind permission from John Wiley & Sons, Ltd

tissue targets required a more articulated protocol, as manipulation and sectioning may induce deformation artifacts that alter the measurements process. To preserve the structural properties of these samples throughout the examination, a snap-freeze technique [29] was used. It consists in rapidly lowering the temperature of samples down to $-70\,^{\circ}$C, by means of dry ice. This technique increases the rigidity of specimens, allowing for sharp and clean slicing with minimum deformation. Targets were sectioned with a cryostat microtome, which allows to perform slicing while keeping the temperature of samples low ($-30\,^{\circ}$C). The depth of incision is defined as the distance from the surface to the bottom of the incision crater (see Fig. 3.8). This was measured through manual segmentation of the microscope images: the depth of incision is estimated contrasting its size in pixels against a reference scalebar.

References

1. M. Thiriet, in *Anatomy and Physiology of the Circulatory and Ventilatory Systems*, ser. Biomathematical and Biomechanical Modeling of the Circulatory and Ventilatory Systems (Springer, 2013)
2. L.S. Mattos, N. Deshpande, G. Barresi, L. Guastini, G. Peretti, A novel computerized surgeon-machine interface for robot-assisted laser phonomicrosurgery. Laryngoscope **124**(8), 1887–1894 (2014)
3. M. Rubinstein, W. Armstrong, Transoral laser microsurgery for laryngeal cancer: A primer and review of laser dosimetry. Lasers Med. Sci. **26**(1), 113–124 (2011)
4. W. Steiner, P. Ambrosch, in *Endoscopic Laser Surgery of the Upper Aerodigestive Tract: with Special Emphasis on Cancer Surgery* (Thieme, 2000)
5. D. Pardo, L. Fichera, D. Caldwell, L. Mattos, in *"Thermal Supervision During Robotic Laser Microsurgery*. 2014 5th IEEE RAS EMBS International Conference on Biomedical Robotics and Biomechatronics (2014), pp. 363–368
6. M. Remacle, G. Lawson, M.-C. Nollevaux, M. Delos, Current state of scanning micromanipulator applications with the carbon dioxide laser. Ann. Otol. Rhinol. Laryngol. **117**(4), 239–244 (2008)
7. M.L. Hinni, A. Ferlito, M.S. Brandwein-Gensler, R.P. Takes, C.E. Silver, W.H. Westra, R.R. Seethala, J.P. Rodrigo, J. Corry, C.R. Bradford, J.L. Hunt, P. Strojan, K.O. Devaney, D.R. Gnepp, D.M. Hartl, L.P. Kowalski, A. Rinaldo, L. Barnes, Surgical margins in head and neck cancer: A contemporary review. Head Neck **35**(9), 1362–1370 (2013)
8. M. Alicandri-Ciufelli, M. Bonali, A. Piccinini, L. Marra, A. Ghidini, E. Cunsolo, A. Maiorana, L. Presutti, P. Conte, Surgical margins in head and neck squamous cell carcinoma: what is close. Eur Arch. Oto-Rhino-Laryngol. **270**(10), 2603–2609 (2013)
9. G. Mannelli, G. Meccariello, A. Deganello, V. Maio, D. Massi, O. Gallo, Impact of low-thermal-injury devices on margin status in laryngeal cancer. An experimental ex vivo study. Oral Oncol. **50**(1), 32–39 (2014)
10. L. Fichera, D. Pardo, L.S. Mattos, in *Virtual Supervision for a Virtual Scalpel*. Proceedings of the 1st Russian-German Conference on Biomedical Engineering (Hanover, 2013)
11. P. Saccomandi, E. Schena, S. Silvestri, Techniques for temperature monitoring during laser-induced thermotherapy: An overview. Int. J. Hyperth. **29**(7), 609–619 (2013)
12. M. Niemz, *Laser-tissue Interactions* (Springer, Berlin, 2004)
13. J.J. Crochet, S.C. Gnyawali, Y. Chen, E.C. Lemley, L.V. Wang, W.R. Chen, Temperature distribution in selective laser-tissue interaction. J. Biomed. Opt. **11**(3), 034(031)–034(031-10) (2006)
14. S. Gnyawali, Y. Chen, F. Wu, K. Bartels, J. Wicksted, H. Liu, C. Sen, W. Chen, Temperature measurement on tissue surface during laser irradiation. Med. Biol. Eng. Comput. **46**(2), 159–168 (2008)
15. J. Jiao, Z. Guo, Thermal interaction of short-pulsed laser focused beams with skin tissues. Phys. Med. Biol. **54**(13), 4225 (2009)
16. E.M. Ahmed, F.J. Barrera, E.A. Early, M.L. Denton, C. Clark, D.K. Sardar, Maxwell's equations-based dynamic laser tissue interaction model. Comput. Biol. Med. **43**(12), 2278–2286 (2013)
17. S. Stopp, D. Svejdar, E. von Kienlin, H. Deppe, T.C. Lueth, A new approach for creating defined geometries by navigated laser ablation based on volumetric 3-d data. IEEE Trans. Biomed. Eng. 1872–1880 (2008)
18. L.A. Kahrs, J. Burgner, T. Klenzner, J. Raczkowsky, J. Schipper, H. Wörn, Planning and simulation of microsurgical laser bone ablation. Int. J. Comput. Assist. Radiol. Surg. **5**(2), 155–162 (2010)
19. B.Y. Leung, P.J. Webster, J.M. Fraser, V.X. Yang, Real-time guidance of thermal and ultrashort pulsed laser ablation in hard tissue using inline coherent imaging. Lasers Surg. Med. **44**(3), 249–256 (2012)

20. E. Bay, X.L. Deán-Ben, G.A. Pang, A. Douplik, D. Razansky, Real-time monitoring of incision profile during laser surgery using shock wave detection. J. Biophotonics (2013)
21. A. Schoob, D. Kundrat, L. Kleingrothe, L. Kahrs, N. Andreff, T. Ortmaier, Tissue surface information for intraoperative incision planning and focus adjustment in laser surgery. Int. J. Comput. Assist. Radiol. Surg. **10**(2), 171–181 (2015)
22. D. Vernon, Cognitive system. Encycl. Comput. Vis. (2012)
23. D. Vernon, G. Metta, G. Sandini, A survey of artificial cognitive systems: Implications for the autonomous development of mental capabilities in computational agents. IEEE Trans. Evol. Comput. **11**(2), 151–180 (2007)
24. M. Mohri, A. Rostamizadeh, A. Talwalkar, *Foundations of Machine Learning*, ser. Adaptive Computation and Machine Learning Series (MIT Press, 2012)
25. L. Mattos, G. Dagnino, G. Becattini, M. Dellepiane, D. Caldwell, "A virtual scalpel system for computer-assisted laser microsurgery," in Intelligent Robots and Systems (IROS). IEEE/RSJ Int. Conf. **2011**, 1359–1365 (2011)
26. D. Pardo, L. Fichera, D. Caldwell, L. Mattos, Learning temperature dynamics on agar-based phantom tissue surface during single point co2 laser exposure. Neural Process. Lett. **42**(1), 55–70 (2015). http://dx.doi.org/10.1007/s11063-014-9389-y
27. S. Rastegar, M.J.C. van Gemert, A.J. Welch, L.J. Hayes, Laser ablation of discs of agar gel. Phys. Med. Biol. **33**(1), 133 (1988)
28. L. Fichera, D. Pardo, P. Illiano, J. Ortiz, D.G. Caldwell, L.S. Mattos, Online estimation of laser incision depth for transoral microsurgery: approach and preliminary evaluation. Int. J. Med. Robot. Comput. Assist. Surg. (2015). http://dx.doi.org/10.1002/rcs.1656
29. M. Shabihkhani, G.M. Lucey, B. Wei, S. Mareninov, J.J. Lou, H.V. Vinters, E.J. Singer, T.F. Cloughesy, W.H. Yong, The procurement, storage, and quality assurance of frozen blood and tissue biospecimens in pathology, biorepository, and biobank settings. Clin. Biochem, **47**(4), 258–266 (2014)

Chapter 4
Learning the Temperature Dynamics During Thermal Laser Ablation

Given the research problem outlined in the previous chapter, here we focus on the development of a methodology to learn the temperature dynamics of tissues subject to thermal laser ablation. Chapter 2 introduced the equations that govern the generation of heat within the tissue during laser irradiation, and the associated increase of temperature. Such relations constitute the starting point of our investigation: based on these, we hypothesize that the superficial temperature of tissue can be modeled, at any given instant in time, as the superposition of Gaussian functions. Nonlinear fitting methods [1] are used to calculate the Gaussian parameters (amplitude, mean and variance) that describe the distribution of temperature at discrete moments in time. The learning problem is formulated as a supervised nonlinear regression, which aims to predict the temporal evolution of the Gaussian parameters.

To understand the viability of the proposed approach we first consider a simple scenario, which does not involve motions of the laser beam. Later in the chapter we present an extension of this methodology to a more general case, to estimate the temperature dynamics produced by a scanning beam.

4.1 Preliminary Considerations

The hypothesis function f defined in Eq. 3.1 estimates the superficial temperature of a slab of tissue subject to laser irradiation, given the applied laser power P, the pulse duration τ, the beam scanning frequency ω_s, and the total laser exposure time t_{exp}. Initial exploration was conducted to better understand the nature of function f and identify an appropriate set of basis functions for the learning task.

Let us consider a simple scenario in which a laser beam, TEM_{00} profile, irradiates a fixed spot on the surface R of a sample of tissue. This scenario is represented in Fig. 4.1. For the sake of simplicity, we assume that the surface of tissue is plain and that the laser beam is normally incident on it. We further assume that the laser is

L. Fichera, *Cognitive Supervision for Robot-Assisted Minimally Invasive Laser Surgery*, Springer Theses, DOI 10.1007/978-3-319-30330-7_4

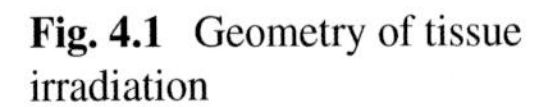
Fig. 4.1 Geometry of tissue irradiation

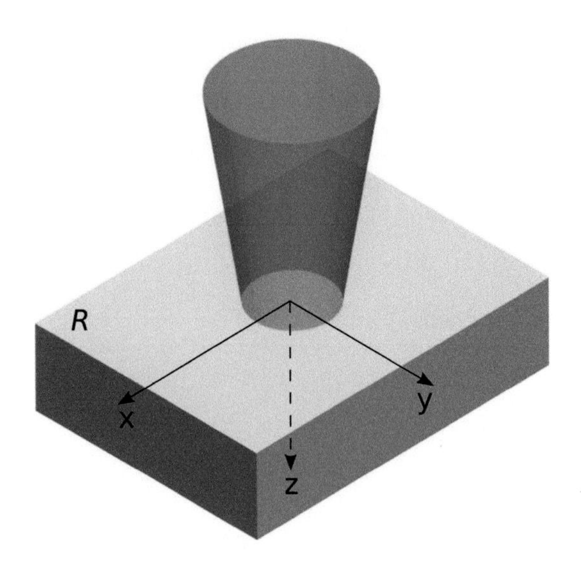

perfectly focused on the surface of tissue. A Cartesian reference frame (x, y, z) is established to describe the tissue geometry, with z being coincident with the beam axis, x and y laying on the R plane. Based on the heat conduction equation (Eq. 2.12), a local variation of tissue temperature occurs, that is modeled as the sum of two distinct contributions: the laser input S $(\mathrm{W} \cdot \mathrm{m}^{-3})$, plus a second-order differential term that accounts for the diffusion of heat within the tissue volume. Although a general formulation for the temporal evolution of temperature $T(t)$ cannot be given analytically, exact solutions can be derived under certain assumptions.

The "1 μs rule" (see Sect. 2.4.2) establishes that the effect of heat diffusion is negligible for short irradiations, i.e. for values of exposure time $t_{exp} < 1\mu\mathrm{s}$ [2]. In this case, the local temperature increase produced by the laser source is:

$$\dot{T} = \frac{1}{\rho c} S. \tag{4.1}$$

Let us recall from Chap. 2 that ρ is the density of tissue $(\mathrm{kg} \cdot \mathrm{m}^{-3})$ and c is its specific heat capacity $(\mathrm{J} \cdot \mathrm{kg}^{-1}\mathrm{K}^{-1})$. Replacing the volumetric energy density S with its definition (Eq. 2.7) yields

$$\dot{T} = \frac{\mu_a}{\rho c} I, \tag{4.2}$$

where μ_a is the absorption coefficient of tissue (m^{-1}). This equation establishes a relation between the temporal derivative of the temperature and the intensity profile I of the laser beam within the tissue volume. Such relation depends on the local values of the absorption coefficient μ_a, tissue density ρ and heat capacity c. Assuming that these coefficients are *isotropic*, i.e. that they are uniform across the tissue sample, it follows that the temperature increase produced by the laser has precisely the same form of the beam intensity, i.e. a Gaussian function. The time dependency of I can be dropped if a constant beam intensity is used. In such a case, Eq. 4.2 has a straightforward solution:

$$T(x, y, z, t) = T_0 + \frac{\mu_a}{\rho c} I(x, y, z)\, t. \tag{4.3}$$

where T_0 is the initial temperature. Imposing $z = 0$ and replacing the intensity I by its definition (Eq. 2.5) we obtain a relation that describe the temporal evolution of the temperature on the surface of tissue:

$$T(x, y, t) = T_0 + \frac{\mu_a}{\rho c} I_0 \exp\left(-\frac{2(x^2 + y^2)}{\omega^2}\right) t. \tag{4.4}$$

We now consider the homogeneous part of the heat conduction equation, that models the temperature variation once the laser source is turned off (i.e. $S = 0$)

$$\dot{T} = \kappa \Delta T, \tag{4.5}$$

where κ is the temperature conductivity of tissue ($m^2 \cdot s^{-1}$). This equation admits solutions of the form[1]

$$T(x, y, z, t) = T_0 + \frac{\alpha \exp\left(-\frac{x^2+y^2+z^2}{4\kappa t}\right)}{(4\pi\kappa t)^{\frac{3}{2}}}, \tag{4.6}$$

with α being an integration constant. From this relation, it follows that the time-dependent distribution of temperature at the tissue surface follows a two-dimensional Gaussian profile:

$$T(x, y, t) = T_0 + \frac{\alpha \exp\left(-\frac{x^2+y^2}{4\kappa t}\right)}{(4\pi\kappa t)^{\frac{3}{2}}}. \tag{4.7}$$

These theoretical results seem to indicate that a combination of Gaussian functions could adequately approximate the superficial temperature of tissue during laser ablation. Nonetheless, in our derivation of Eqs. 4.4 and 4.7, we have used many assumptions that certainly do not hold in the case of laser ablation. The ablation process induces disruptive modifications in the tissue both at the mechanical and physical levels (alterations in the density, absorption and thermal conductivity), whereas the calculations above assume a fixed tissue geometry and isotropic conditions. Furthermore, the CO_2 lasers used in clinical practice present pulse durations $\tau \geq 1\mu s$: for these durations the effects of heat diffusion can no longer be neglected and, as it was pointed out earlier, the solution $T(t)$ must be extracted using numerical approximation methods. Based on these considerations, it is unclear whether a

[1] A proof is given in Appendix B.

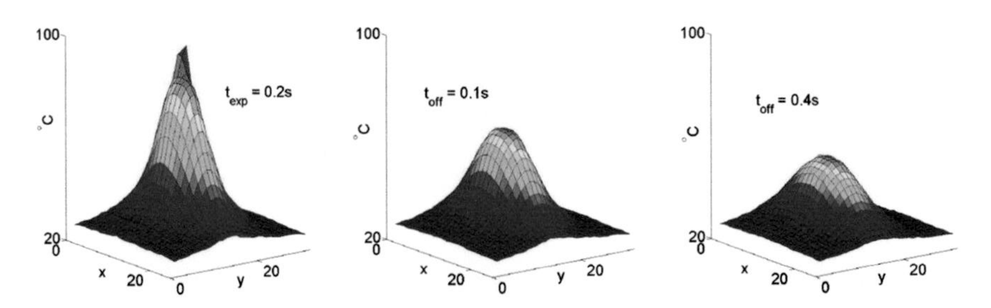

Fig. 4.2 Temperature distribution captured at different moments of the experiment. **a** Laser exposed for $t_{exp} = 0.2$ s, **b** After exposure, laser is turned off ($t_{off} = 0.1$ s) and **c** $t_{off} = 0.4$ s. Reproduced from [3] with kind permission from Springer Science+Business Media

Gaussian model is adequate for the approximation of the superficial tissue temperature T. To better understand the validity of this hypothesis, we performed a series of preliminary laser experiments.

Agar-based gel phantoms were irradiated with a CO_2 laser source (beam waist $\omega_s = 250$ μm), using an exposure time $t_{exp} = 0.2$ s. The superficial temperature was captured with an infrared thermal camera, at a rate of 100 Hz. This sensor provides a sequence of images that contains the values of temperature for a predefined continuous rectangular plane S centered at the point of laser incision. Before being irradiated, the samples were kept at room temperature (~25 °C) for 10 min. The sequence in Fig. 4.2 shows typical temperature profiles obtained during the trials: the xy plane of the plot corresponds to the surface of the tissue, values of temperature have been plotted in the z-axis. Each pixel represents the temperature value (°C) of an area that covers $0.177 \times 0.177\,\text{mm}^2$.

Visual analysis of the plots in Fig. 4.2 indicates that the superficial temperature of tissue can be reasonably assumed to have a Gaussian distribution. Temperature spikes are observed during laser irradiation, next to the peak of the Gaussian surface. These might be produced by the expulsion of hot plume from the ablation site.

4.2 Single-Point Ablation

In this section we derive a methodology to learn the temporal evolution of tissue temperature during single-point laser ablation. Let $T(R, k) \in \mathbb{R}^{m \times n}$ be the two-dimensional matrix representing the temperature of R at the discrete time step k, assuming that $k = 0$ coincides with the time instant when the interaction starts. The temperature of any point $x, y \in R$ will be given by the (i, j)-element of the matrix, following the quantizations,

$$i = \left\lceil \frac{y}{\Delta_y} \right\rceil, j = \left\lceil \frac{x}{\Delta_x} \right\rceil \tag{4.8}$$

where $\Delta_y = Y/m$, $\Delta_x = X/n$, and the $\lceil \cdot \rceil$ notation expresses the ceil function, i.e., *the smallest integer not less than.*

Temperature of the surface is not uniform and changes with time, i.e.,

$$T(R, k) = f(x, y, k). \tag{4.9}$$

where $(x, y) \in R$ correspond to the pixel coordinates of any point on the surface. Based on the ideas presented in the previous section, we define a hypothesis function given by a Gaussian function with variable parameters,

$$T(R, k) = A(k) \exp\left(-\left(\frac{(x - \mu_x(k))^2}{2\sigma_x^2(k)} + \frac{(y - \mu_y(k))^2}{2\sigma_y^2(k)}\right)\right) \tag{4.10}$$

where A represents the amplitude σ_x and σ_y the spatial spreads of the Gaussian, and μ_x, μ_y the center of the function. Note that this hypothesis assumes symmetry with respect to the xy axis in the energy distribution delivered by the laser. Thus, this model can represent elliptical temperature profiles without rotation.

4.2.1 *Fitting a Gaussian Function*

A thermal camera is used to collect data for the learning task. At each time step, this provides a set of points $\left\{(x, y)^i, T^i\right\}_{i=1}^{m \times n}$ points from which the vector of parameters $\theta(k) = \left[A, \sigma_x^2, \sigma_y^2, \mu_x, \mu_y\right]$ needs to be estimated. A common approach is to use a linear version of the model, which is obtained by applying a logarithmic operator to both sides of the equation,

$$\log T = \alpha_0 + \alpha_1 x + \alpha_2 y + \alpha_3 x^2 + \alpha_4 y^2. \tag{4.11}$$

Hence, the nonlinear regression for (4.10) is transformed into a linear regression with *meta parameters*, $\alpha \in \mathbb{R}^5$ [4]. The elements of θ are then given by,

$$\begin{aligned} \sigma_x^2 &= -(2\alpha_4)^{-1} & , \ \sigma_y^2 &= -(2\alpha_3)^{-1} \\ \mu_x &= \alpha_2 \sigma_x^2 & , \ \mu_y &= \alpha_1 \sigma_y^2 \\ A &= \exp\left(\alpha_0 + \frac{\mu_x^2}{2\sigma_x^2} + \frac{\mu_y^2}{2\sigma_y^2}\right). \end{aligned} \tag{4.12}$$

A least square regression can then be applied to fit the sensor data in (4.11). Nevertheless, given that there is more data in the tail of the Gaussian than in the bell, weighting the sample points by its correspondent estimation balance the influence of the entire data set during the minimization of the sum of square errors. This is known as weighted least-square minimization (see [5]).

4.2.2 Meta-Parameters Dynamics

Fitting the hypothesis function (4.10) to the data captured during a real laser exposure provides a different vector of parameters for each time step. Figure 4.2 shows data corresponding to different times during laser exposure. In order to estimate the temperature at any point and time using such model a lookup table of hundreds of vectors of parameters would be required.

We propose to investigate a function describing the dynamics of the parameters $\theta(k)$, i.e. given the initial value $\theta(0)$ and an input $u(k)$ signal, the evolution of such parameters can be described using,

$$\theta_i(k+1) = h(\theta_i(k), \theta_i(0), u(k)), \tag{4.13}$$

where $u(k)$ may assume one of the following values:

$$u(k) = \begin{cases} 1 \; \textit{laser on/heating} \\ 0 \; \textit{laser off/cooling} \end{cases} \tag{4.14}$$

At the same time, it is important to note that the sequence of Gaussian parameters include errors from the noise in the raw data. Furthermore, these errors are propagated by the use of the logarithmic linear regression method and by the mapping from the meta parameters in (4.12). This is especially true for the amplitude (A), which is derived from a nonlinear function of the entire vector of meta parameters. To prevent the propagation of noise from further affecting the quality of the estimation (i.e., the quality of h) we propose to model the evolution of the meta parameters, i.e.,

$$\alpha(k+1) = g(\alpha(k), \alpha(0), u(k)). \tag{4.15}$$

The quality of g in (4.15) is expected to be better than the one of h in (4.13), given the level of noise in the respective data set.

4.2.3 Experiments

This section describes the experiments performed to capture the data to learn and validate the model. Single spot laser radiations on agar-based phantom tissue were produced using a CO_2 laser system. Temperature of the surface is captured continuously during laser exposure plus a proportional time after the laser is turning off in order to capture the cooling down process. Exposure time was precisely controlled with a computerized system.

Experiment Procedure

Each experiment consisted in firing a CO_2 Continuous Wave (CW) beam at constant power (P = 3W) on the flat surface of a tissue phantom. A different agar sample was used for each experiment. Samples were stored in a refrigerated bath and taken out at room temperature (~25 °C) 10 min before the experiment. The exposure time of each experiment was electronically controlled and an independent sequence of thermal images was recorded. A total of 26 experiments were conducted, varying the exposure time from $t_{exp} = 2.0$ s to $t_{exp} = 4.5$ s with increments of 0.1 s.

Data Sets

To solve the approximation problems formulated in Sects. 4.2.1 and 4.2.2 different data sets were created. Here we describe the structure and the content of these sets.

The former is a fitting problem, it aims to find the optimal Gaussian parameters θ_k that represent the superficial temperature at any time step k. This problem was applied to all of the thermal video frames captured during the laser experiments. During each experiment, a total of $(t_{exp} + t_{off}) \times 100$ frames were captured, each being a matrix with $l = m \times n = 3402$ values of temperature. Frames taken both during the laser exposure and the cooling off phase were considered.

Every experiment corresponds to a sequence of fitted Gaussian parameters θ_k, each representing the time evolution of temperature. These sequences are used to generate the input ($\mathbf{x}$) and output ($\mathbf{y}$) vectors required to learn function described in Eq. 4.13:

$$\mathbf{x} = [\theta_k^i, u_k^i] \tag{4.16}$$

$$\mathbf{y} = [\theta_{k+1}^i]. \tag{4.17}$$

Note that the input incorporates the laser input term u_k^i, which is required to estimate the variation of the values of parameters.

4.2.4 Results

Here we present the results for the Gaussians fitting of the single thermal images, the models obtained after learning the meta parameter dynamics and the temperature prediction that resulted from this data.

Gaussian Fitting

As mentioned in the previous section, a total of $(t_{exp} + t_{off}) \times 100$ Gaussians are approximated. Figure 4.3 shows an example data set and the corresponding

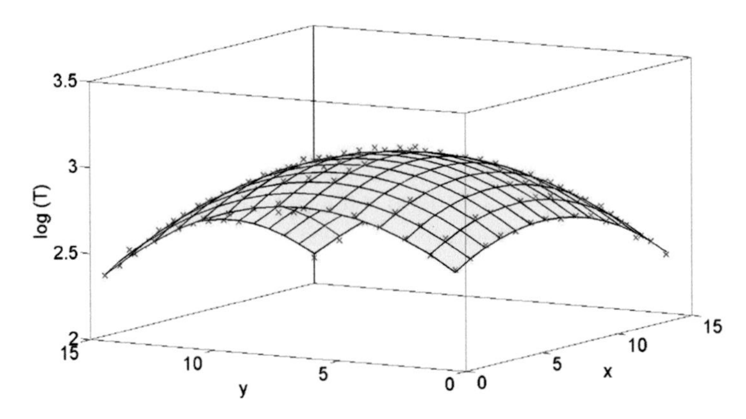

Fig. 4.3 The surface represents the linear regression obtained for input space (x, y) mapping to $z = \log(T)$, using the sensor data (*red* markers). Note that this is not the geometrical representation of the tissue. Reproduced from [3] with kind permission from Springer Science+Business Media

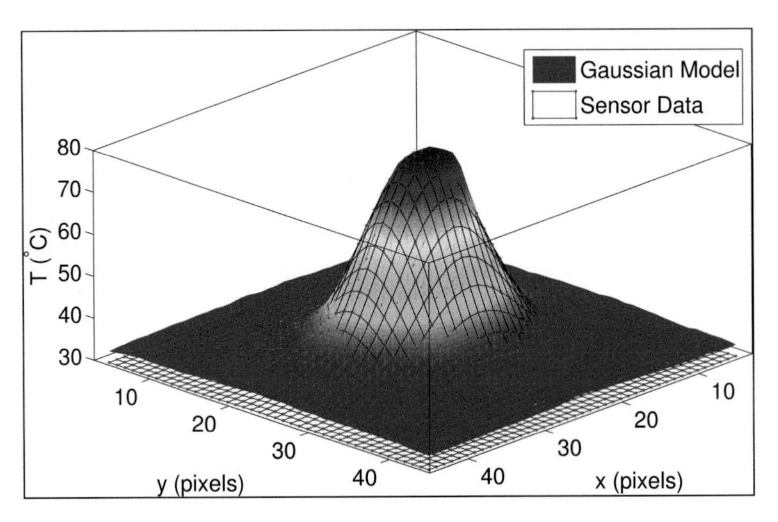

Fig. 4.4 Weighted least *square* estimation of the Gaussian model for a single time step. Corresponding parameters are $\mu = [9.27 \;\; 7.67]$, $\sigma^2 = [26.5 \;\; 15.78]$ and $A = 60.6457$, Approximation error (mse) = 0.0156. Reproduced from [3] with kind permission from Springer Science+Business Media

logarithmic linear regression. Figure 4.4 shows the result of fitting the thermal imaging sensor data to the hypothesis function in Eq. (4.10). The approximation error varies depending on the time of exposure. The temporal evolution of the normalized and root mean squared errors are presented in Fig. 4.6. It can be observed that the approximation of most of the frames present relatively low errors. Nonetheless, for the initial frames the approximation has high values of normalized mean square error (nMSE), indicating that the assumption of Gaussian shape is not completely verified. On the other hand, these frames present only a few Celsius of absolute average error

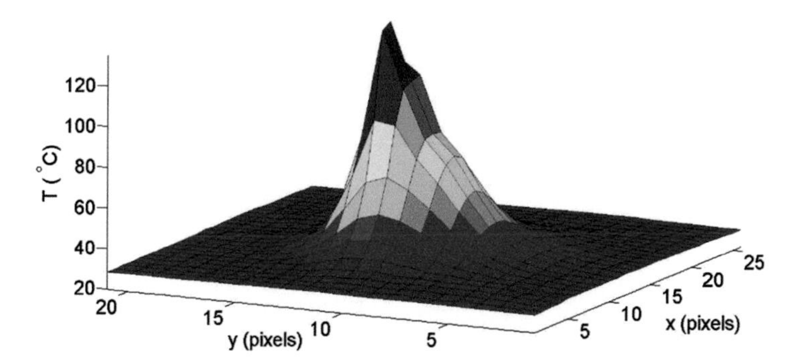

Fig. 4.5 Initial frames include high peaks of temperature that are not modeled by the Gaussian function. The peak points correspond to ablated tissue. Reproduced from [3] with kind permission from Springer Science+Business Media

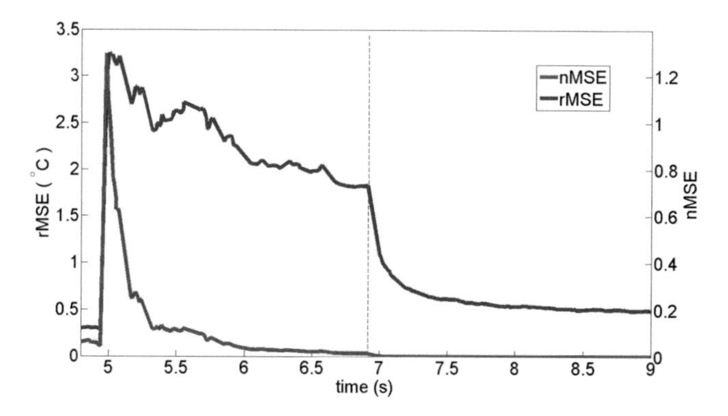

Fig. 4.6 Gaussian function approximation error for a complete experiment. RMSE (*blue*) and nMSE (*red*) changes depending on the stage of the interaction. The nMSE tends to zero after the initial time steps. Reproduced from [3] with kind permission from Springer Science+Business Media

(RMSE). Visual analysis of the initial frames reveals that these errors are largely due to the presence of the temperature peaks at the center of the beam (Fig. 4.5). These peaks are values of temperature at the center of the beam that last only one time step ($\Delta t = 0.01$ s) and we consider as noise. As we have commented earlier in this chapter, these peaks might have the following physical explanation, i.e. that they correspond to the expulsion of material from the ablation site—for which, therefore, temperature monitoring is not relevant.

Temporal Evolution of the Gaussian Parameters

Figure 4.7 shows the temporal evolution of the Gaussian parameters A, σ_x^2, σ_y^2 during a total exposure time and laser power similar to those used in laryngeal surgery

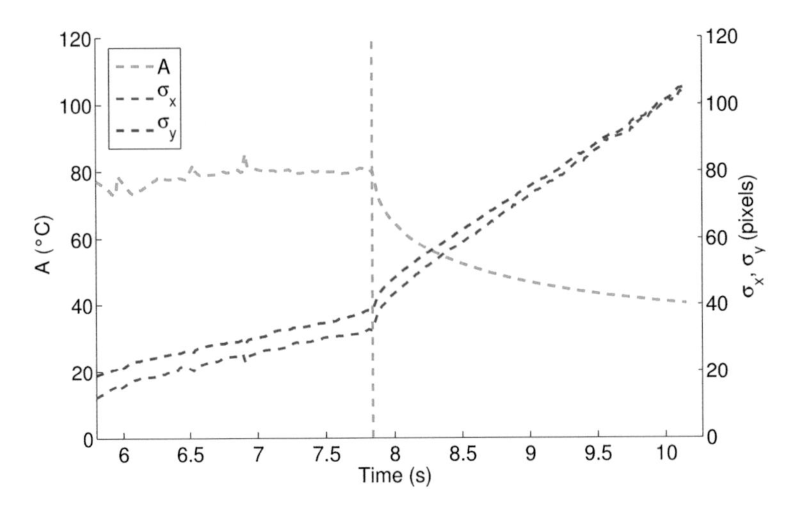

Fig. 4.7 Time evolution of the Gaussian parameters (A, σ_x, σ_y) during a $t_{exp} = 2\,\text{s}$ interaction ($t_0 = 5.8\,\text{s}$, $t_f = 7.8\,\text{s}$). It includes the heating and cooling phases. Reproduced from [3] with kind permission from Springer Science+Business Media

($P = 3.0$ W, $t_{exp} = 2\,\text{s}$). As expected, the parameters evolve differently when the laser is turned on. Different versions of Eq. (4.13) need to be learned to model both behaviors (heating, cooling) although the underlying structure of the hypothesis remains the same.

During laser exposure the amplitude of the Gaussian remains rather constant (Fig. 4.7), while the spread of the temperature over the tissue clearly increases. The instantaneous peaks of temperature observed in the center of the beam are naturally filtered by the linear regression.

When the laser is turned off the maximum temperature decreases and the rate of change of the variance increases. This is consistent with the analytic solution of the (homogeneous) heat transfer equation, where the amplitude of the function is inversely proportional to the square root of time, while the variance is proportional to it [2]. It can also be observed that the behavior of σ_x^2 and σ_y^2 are similar but not exactly the same: although the energy density produced by our laser is cylindrically symmetric (TEM_{00}), the orientation of the camera with respect to the target introduces a perspective deformation. This deformation was kept under control maintaining the position of the camera constant throughout the experiments. The sequence of means (μ_x, μ_y) is not showed as it remain almost constant throughout the experiment.

Dynamics of the Metaparameters

The exponential time evolution shown by the meta parameters in Fig. 4.8 suggests a first order dynamics for g of the form,

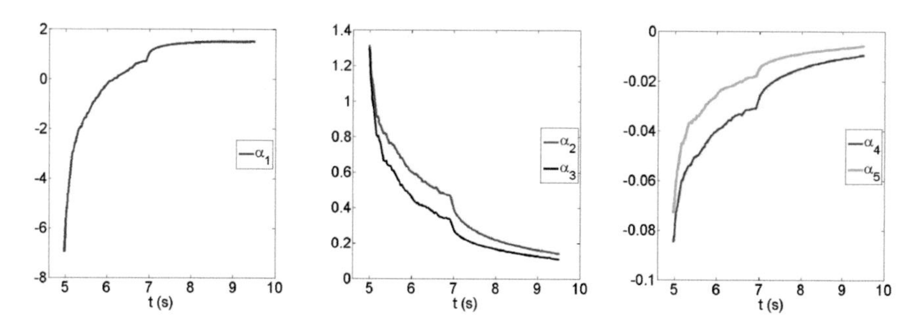

Fig. 4.8 Meta parameters time evolution α_1 (*blue*), α_2 (*red*), α_3 (*black*), α_4 (*green*), α_5 (*magenta*). Reproduced from [3] with kind permission from Springer Science+Business Media

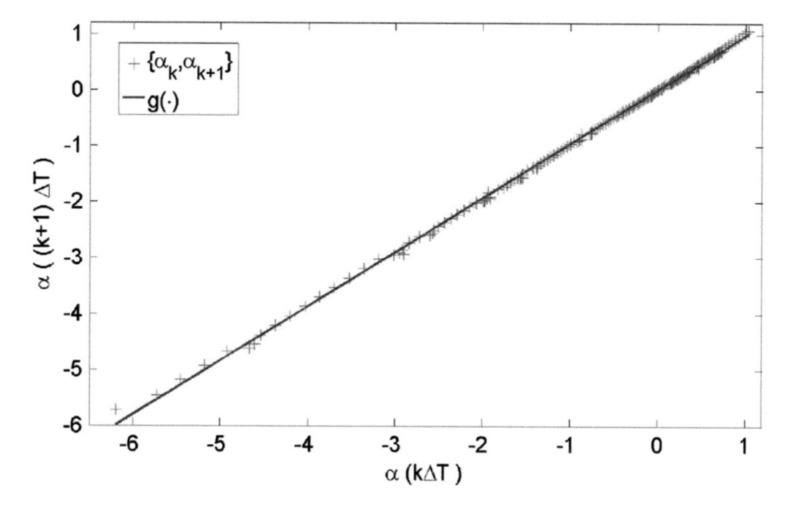

Fig. 4.9 First order dynamics in the meta parameter space $\alpha(k), \alpha(k+1)$. Reproduced from [3] with kind permission from Springer Science+Business Media

$$
\begin{aligned}
\alpha(k+1) &= g(\alpha(k), \alpha(0)) \\
\alpha(k+1) &= C_1\alpha(k) + C_0
\end{aligned}
\tag{4.18}
$$

where C_1 and C_0 can be extracted with a simple polynomial regression between $\alpha(k+1)$ and $\alpha(k)$, as shown in Fig. 4.9. Simplified plots of the discrete dynamics of the meta parameters (both for heating and cooling models) are shown for completeness in Fig. 4.10. The resulting model parameters (C_0, C_1) are presented in Table 4.1.

Temperature Estimation

The estimation of temperature only requires the initial state of the meta parameters vector, then the recursion in (4.18) evolves with the activation/deactivation of the

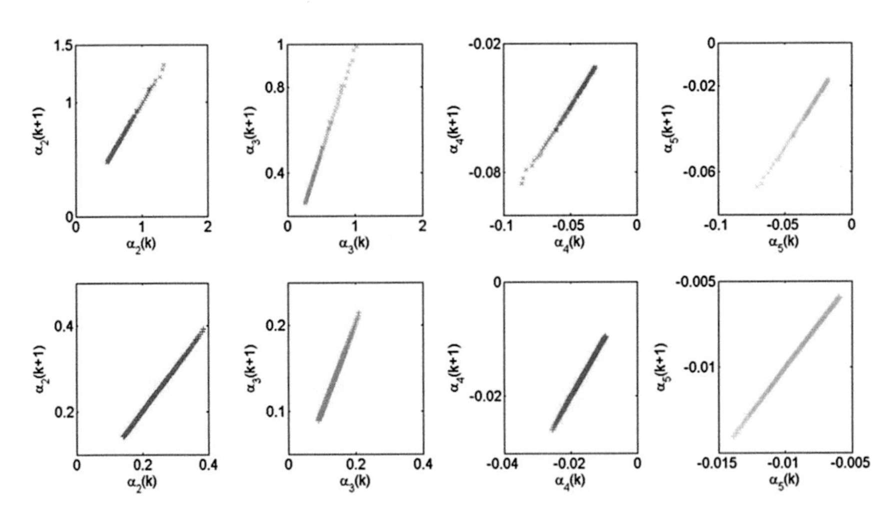

Fig. 4.10 Discrete dynamics of the meta parameters ($\alpha_i \; i = 1, 2, 3, 4$). Both models are shown; 'laser on/heating' (*first row*) and 'laser off/cooling' (*second row*). Reproduced from [3] with kind permission from Springer Science+Business Media

Table 4.1 Table of constants for the meta parameters linear dynamics for both models: heating (laser on) and cooling (laser off)

α	$C0_{on}$	$C1_{on}$	$C0_{off}$	$C1_{off}$
1	0.9637	0.0333	0.9557	0.0772
2	0.9705	0.0155	0.9869	0.0019
3	0.9646	0.0108	0.9864	0.0012
4	0.9716	–0.0010	0.9876	–0.0001
5	0.9649	–0.0007	0.9879	–0.0001

Reproduced from [3] with kind permission from Springer Science+Business Media

laser input. The Gaussian parameters and therefore the surface temperature can be estimated at any time of interest. Figure 4.11 shows the comparison between the real time change of the meta parameters and that obtained with the recursion. Figure 4.12 shows an example of surface temperature reconstruction (nMSE = 0.0137).

4.2.5 Discussion

The model presented in this section is able to predict temperature of the surface of tissue gel phantoms during single point CO_2 laser ablation. The modeling process takes advantage of the Gaussian structure of the data and here we explain such structure analyzing the shape of the energy spatial profile in the laser beam.

Although the hypothesis function allows us to model elliptical shapes for the Gaussian, it assumes that it is not rotated. Due to the physical location of the sensor

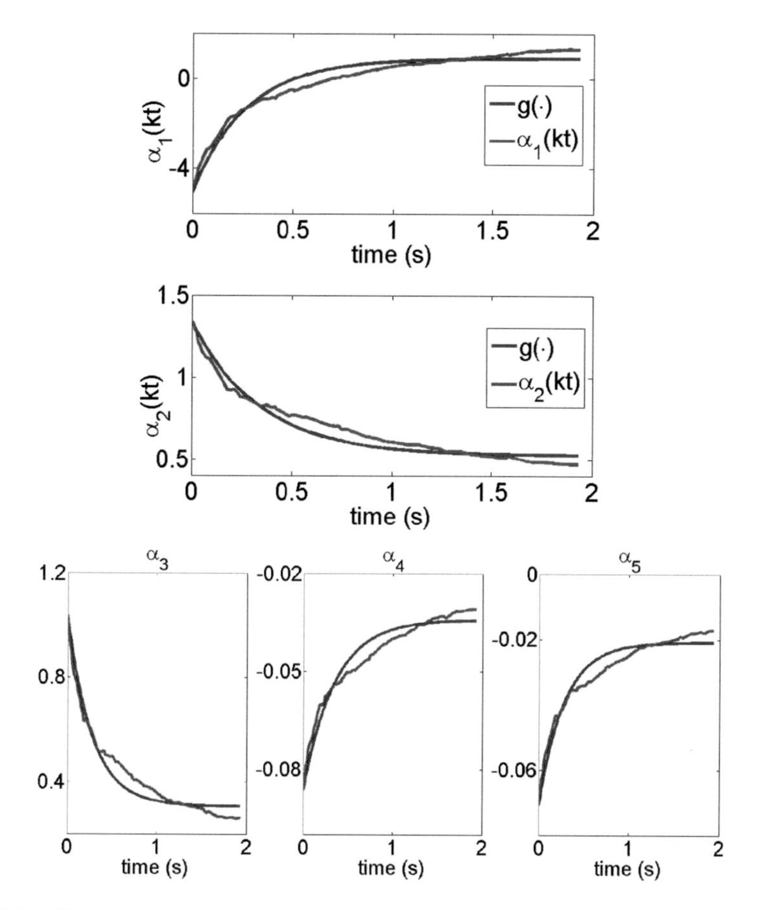

Fig. 4.11 Time evolution of the meta parameters (α_i). Learned dynamics (*blue*) extracted from data (*red*). Reproduced from [3] with kind permission from Springer Science+Business Media

some perspective was generated and data captured by the thermal camera showed that minor rotation were present. The model can be augmented, including parameters for the xy distribution of temperature, improving the fitting error. This fitting error may also be improved using an iterative method for Gaussian approximation [5].

The assumption that the dynamics of the meta parameters α is easier to model than the one of the Gaussian parameters θ can be observed in Fig. 4.13, where the sequence of values for the first element of both sets is shown. It can be seen that the pattern of α_1 can be described using a first order dynamics, whereas that of θ_1 is much more complicated to describe.

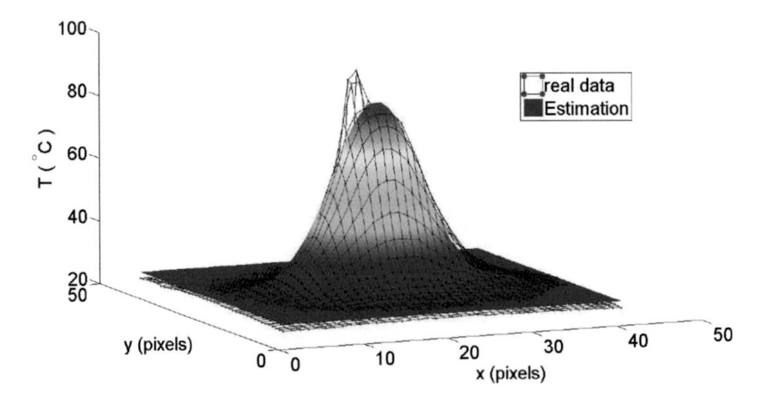

Fig. 4.12 Temperature reconstruction. At a given time during laser exposure (t_{exp} = 1.92) the temperature of the surface is estimated using the evolution of the meta parameters with nMSE = 0.0137. Reproduced from [3] with kind permission from Springer Science+Business Media

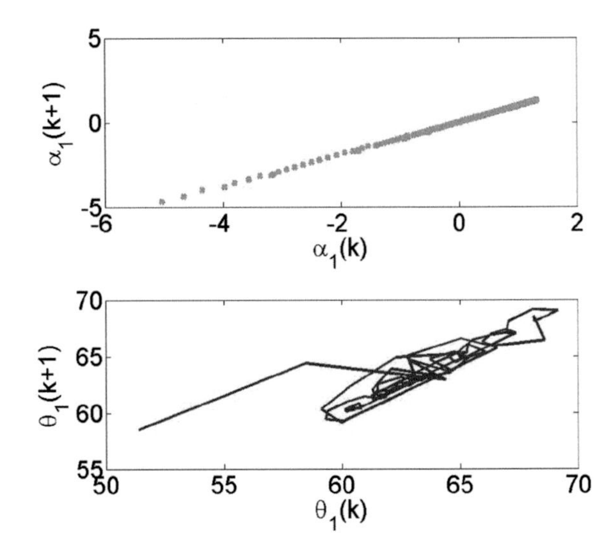

Fig. 4.13 Discrete dynamics of the first element of the meta parameter vector (α_1) as well as of the Gaussian parameter (θ_1). The pattern of $\alpha_1(k)$ can be modeled with a first order system. Reproduced from [3] with kind permission from Springer Science+Business Media

4.3 Temperature Dynamics During Laser Scanning

We now seek to extend our modeling methodology to the more general case of tissue ablation by means of a scanning laser beam. The motion of the laser beam directly affects the time-dependent energy density S, thus determining a different thermal response. Evidence presented so far in this chapter indicates that, in the case of single point ablation, the temperature $T(t)$ on the surface of tissue may be modeled by a single Gaussian function with time-varying parameters. The use of a moving laser beam imposes the use of a different model, whose structure is determined experimentally, from the analysis of data collected during preliminary laser trials.

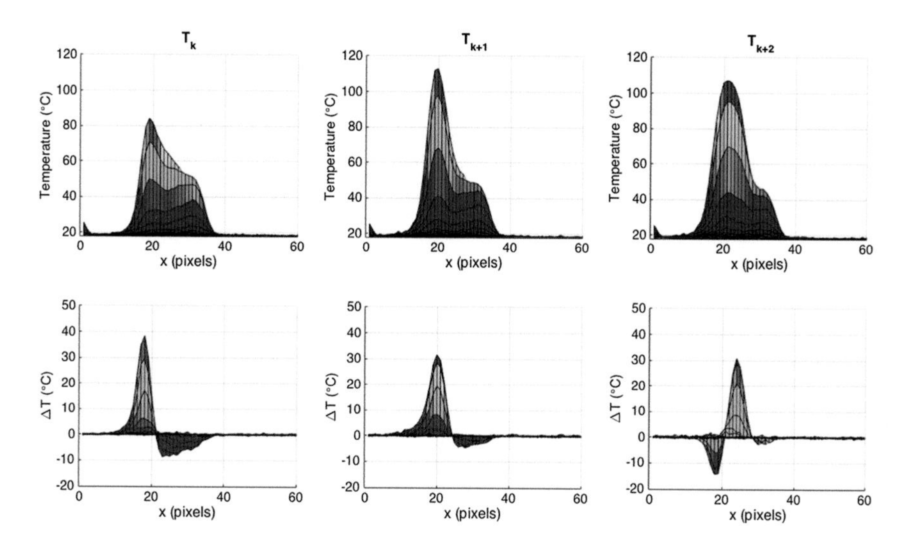

Fig. 4.14 *First row* Tissue temperature profile during computer controlled incision ($l = 0.3$ mm, $w = 10$ Hz). Although the Gaussian distribution of the energy in the laser beam is present, the profile does not show any particular pattern as it grows in time. *Second row* Temporal change on temperature $\Delta T = T(R, k+1) - T(R, k-1)$. Adapted from [6]

Incisions were created on ex-vivo chicken muscle tissue samples, by means of a laser scanning system (described in Sect. 3.6.1). The laser beam is moved repeatedly along a line of length ($l = 4.6$ mm), during certain exposure time (t_{exp}). The motion of the laser scans the complete line at a configurable velocity and oscillatory frequency (ω_s). Therefore, the number of times the laser scans the incision is given by $\eta = t_{exp}/\omega_s$. The period of time the tissue is exposed to the laser is uniformly distributed along the incision line.

Examples of the superficial temperature profile for different times k of the process $T(R, k)$ are shown in the first row of Fig. 4.14. With the aim of reducing the problem complexity, we take the y axis to be coincident with the laser scanning trajectory. We further assume symmetry with respect to the incision line, thus only the temperature along the x axis is shown. The Gaussian-shaped contribution of the laser input S can be visually recognized in the correspondence of the temperature peaks. Nonetheless, as the beam moves along the incision, the temperature profile does not seem to present any specific pattern as it evolves in time.

The second row of Fig. 4.14 shows the temperature increments for the corresponding exposure time. These sequence suggests that the temporal increment of the temperature $\Delta T(k) = T(R, k+1) - T(R, k)$ could be described as a set of Gaussian functions with centers along the incision line. The positive part of ΔT seems always amenable to be described by a single Gaussian, while the negative part shows diverse conformations. Based on the heat conduction equation (2.12), the positive corresponds to the thermal effects of the input S plus the heat exchange with underlying and surrounding tissue. Thus, the center of this Gaussian is expected to move together with the laser beam along the incision. The negative part of ΔT constitutes the effects of heat diffusion within tissue, which is modeled by the homogeneous part of the heat conduction equation (Eq. 4.5) by a second-order differential term. This indicates that the shape of the negative part should contain higher order differences of $T(R,k)$.

Based on these observations, we theorize that the function describing the temperature of the surface at each frame of the process can be approximated as a sum of Gaussian functions,

$$T(R,k) = \sum_{i=1}^{p} \exp(x, y, a_i, \sigma_i, \mu_i) \tag{4.19}$$

where p is the total number of Gaussians and a_i, μ_i and σ_i are the corresponding amplitude, mean and covariance. Nonlinear least square fitting regression [1] can be applied to fit (4.19) to the experimental data.

4.3.1 *Experiments*

Ex-vivo chicken muscle tissue is used as target for the incision trials. Incision length ($l = 4.6$ mm/25 pixels) and scanning frequency (w $= 10$ Hz) are kept constant. Laser power ($P = 3$ W), and exposure mode (Continuous Wave) were also configured. Total exposure time is set to $t_{exp} = 1.0$ s.

4.3.2 *Results*

The x-axis is aligned with the incision line and the spatial distribution of the temperature is assumed to be symmetric with respect to the y-axis. Here we compare the quality of the model for different values of p. Based on the knowledge provided by (Eq. 2.12), we may hypothesize that the number of Gaussians required for the model is $p = 4$. Nevertheless here we compare the models for different values of p.

For the simplified case of one-dimensional distribution of temperature, the temperature on the incision line $T_k(x)$ is defined by the function

$$T_k(x) \approx \sum_{i=1}^{p} \exp(x, \mu_i, \sigma_i) \tag{4.20}$$

Each experiment is composed by 100 data sets ($t_{exp} = 1.0$ s, $\Delta t = 0.01$ s). The number of input-output pairs per data set is given by the width (in pixels) of the area of interest. Thus, the model is composed by a total of 100 regressions, each one is obtained using $m = 60$ data pairs $\{x_j, T_j\}_{j=1}^{m}$. Figure 4.16 shows three examples of function approximated.

Table 4.2 Regression results analysis: Mean square error (MSE) for $n = 100$ regressions

p	MSE_{max}	MSE_{min}	Mean	Median	Q3–Q1
3	17.57	0.24	3.42	2.93	2.03
4	6.87	0.21	2.31	1.99	1.72
5	4.67	0.23	1.85	1.63	1.35

Adapted from [6]

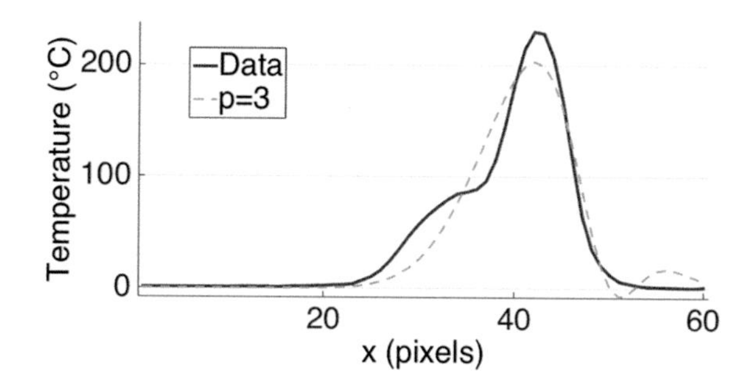

Fig. 4.15 Regression result ($p = 3$). Real temperature is also shown. Adapted from [6]

Modeling Error

The output of the regression at each time step is a vector of parameters (amplitudes, means and standard deviation), $\theta_k = [a_k, \mu_k, \sigma_k]$, where $a, \mu, \sigma \in \mathbb{R}^p$. Each data set generates an approximation error, i.e., it is variable along the experiment. The mean square error (MSE) is analyzed to compare the quality of the model for different values of $p = 3, 4, 5$. Table 4.2 summarizes the information about the variability of the regression error along the experiment, including maximum, minimum, mean, median and interquartile range. It can be seen that the model fits better when using more Gaussians: $p = 4$ performs better than $p = 3$, while not significant improvements can be observed by increasing the number of basis functions to $p = 5$. With $p = 4$, the regression achieves an accuracy (Root-Mean-Square Error) of 1.52 °C, with the largest error ($RMSE_{max}$) being 2.62 °C. Figure 4.15 shows the temperature estimation when modeling with few Gaussian basis functions. On the other hand, Fig. 4.16 shows three examples of regressions with $p = 4$. Different forms of temperature profile are shown.

4.3.3 *Model Validation*

Based on the analysis presented above, a model using $p = 4$ is selected to estimate the temperature dynamics during laser exposure. A total of 12 parameters for each time step are used for prediction.

In order to validate the model, a new experiment is performed and thermal data is captured while the model estimates the temperature profile. Validation error is

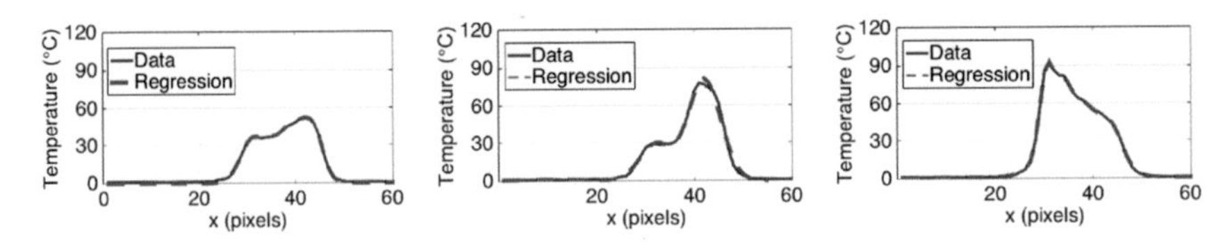

Fig. 4.16 Temperature profile at different stages of the incision. Continuous line (*solid blue line*) shows data collected from experiments, dash line (*red*) shows the result of the regression $p = 4$. Adapted from [6]

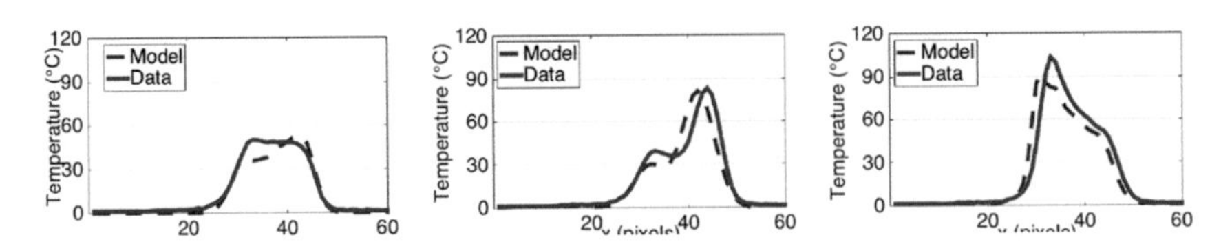

Fig. 4.17 Validation experiments. Sensor data (*solid blue line*) and the corresponding temperature predicted by the model (*dashed violet line*). Adapted from [6]

Table 4.3 Validation results analysis: Mean square error (MSE) for $p = 4$ and $n = 100$ regressions

MSE_{max}	MSE_{min}	Mean	Median	Q3–Q1
19.27	4.44	12.52	13.41	10.34

Adapted from [6]

computed pixel-wise during $t_{exp} = 1$ s. Figure 4.17 shows the real temperature profile for the validation experiment and the resulted temperature estimation (for the same time steps used in Fig. 4.16). It can be observed that the new experiment slightly varies with respect to the learning data set. This causes a relatively high pixel-wise error, as presented in Table 4.3.

Nevertheless, the range and distribution of the temperature is effectively estimated at each time step. In order to illustrate this, a comparison between the maximum value at each time step is shown in Fig. 4.18. It can be observed that the model captures the dynamics of the temperature change. The shape of the temperature profile is compared by computing the area under the curve at each time step, also shown in Fig. 4.18. It can be observed that the model is able to effectively estimate the thermal state of the tissue surface.

4.3.4 Discussion

The experimental evidence presented in this section indicates that statistical learning enables the creation of models capable of reliably estimating tissue temperature

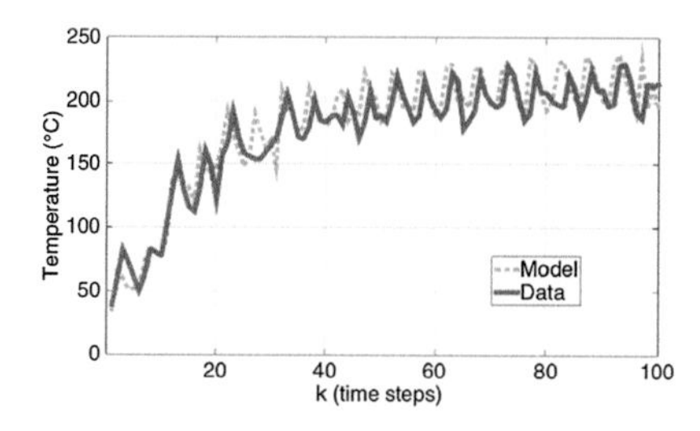

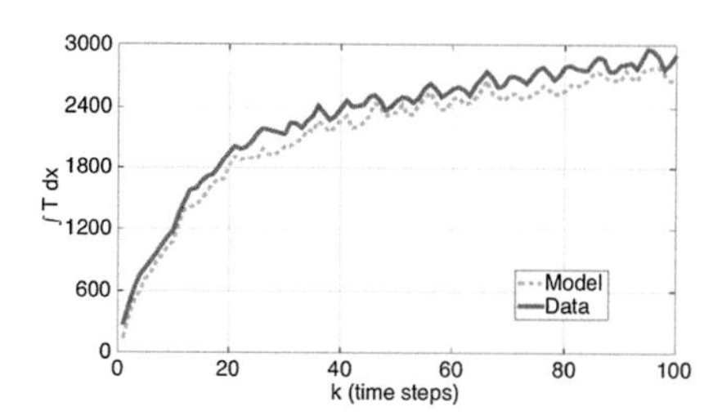

Fig. 4.18 Validation experiment. Maximum values of temperature for each time step are presented (*top*). The integral of the area under the curve for each time step is also presented (*bottom*). Adapted from [6]

variations during laser incisions. These models are straightforward to implement in a surgical setup, as they do not require any additional sensing device.

The model presented here was derived on ex-vivo chicken muscle tissue. Although not representative of the variety of tissues that are encountered during a laryngeal intervention [7], these targets present the behavior of a generic soft tissue, allowing to prove the proposed concept. Our modeling study does not explicitly take into account heat transfer mechanisms typical of living tissues, e.g. blood perfusion. Nonetheless, the contribution of these mechanisms to the local variation of temperature is neglectable in first approximation [2].

In Chap. 6, we shall describe the integration of this model in an experimental surgical platform. Activation and deactivation of the model will be synchronized with the laser activation, allowing online estimation of the temperature of the tissue surface.

References

1. D. Bates, D. Watts, in *Nonlinear Regression Analysis and Its Applications*, ser. Wiley Series in Probability and Statistics (Wiley, 2007)
2. M. Niemz, *Laser-tissue Interactions* (Springer, Berlin, 2004)

3. D. Pardo, L. Fichera, D. Caldwell, L. Mattos, Learning temperature dynamics on agar-based phantom tissue surface during single point co_2 laser exposure. Neural Process. Lett. **42**(1), 55–70 (2015). http://dx.doi.org/10.1007/s11063-014-9389-y
4. R.A. Caruana, R.B. Searle, T. Heller, S.I. Shupack, Fast algorithm for the resolution of spectra. Anal. Chem. **58**(6), 1162–1167 (1986)
5. H. Guo, A simple algorithm for fitting a gaussian function. IEEE Sig. Process. Mag. **28**(5), 134–137 (2011)
6. D. Pardo, L. Fichera, D. Caldwell, L. Mattos, in *Thermal Supervision During Robotic Laser Microsurgery*. 2014 5th IEEE RAS EMBS International Conference on Biomedical Robotics and Biomechatronics (2014), pp. 363–368
7. S.L. Jacques, Optical properties of biological tissues: a review. Phys. Med. Biol. **58**(11), R37 (2013)

Chapter 5
Modeling the Laser Ablation Process

This chapter focuses on the problem of modeling the laser ablation process from a geometrical point of view. The objective is to create a model capable of describing the laser incision depth based on the knowledge of the laser parameters and inputs. The discussion starts with a statement of the problem, which is defined in terms of a supervised regression. Our approach is compared with existing heuristic models for the prediction of ablation depth.

Multiple parameters influence the laser ablation process. With regard to the surgical equipment in use today, these are laser power, delivery mode, pulse duration, scanning frequency. To fully understand the effects of these parameters, first we report on controlled experiments where only one parameter at a time is modified and the resulting depth of incision is examined.

The incision depth is modeled as a function of the laser exposure time. The inverse model is also extracted, which allows to calculate the exposure time required to reach a given incision depth. This inverse model is used in a feed forward setting, to prove the concept of the automatic incision of soft tissue. In addition, we demonstrate how the model can be used to implement the automatic ablation of entire volumes of tissue, through the superposition of controlled laser incisions. The chapter is concluded by a discussion of the findings for the depth estimation model, whose accuracy is considered from a clinical perspective.

5.1 Preliminary Considerations

The hypothesis formulated in Sect. 3.4 seeks to find a function f that relates the depth of the etch created by thermal laser ablation with the laser parameters. The geometry of the problem is illustrated in Fig. 5.1, which shows the creation of an incision by means of laser scans on a tissue target. The same simplifying assumptions used for temperature modeling are made here, i.e. that the slab of tissue presents a flat surface and that the laser is normally incident with respect to it. Without any loss of generality, here we restrict the motion of the laser to a straight line l, facilitating

L. Fichera, *Cognitive Supervision for Robot-Assisted Minimally Invasive Laser Surgery*, Springer Theses, DOI 10.1007/978-3-319-30330-7_5

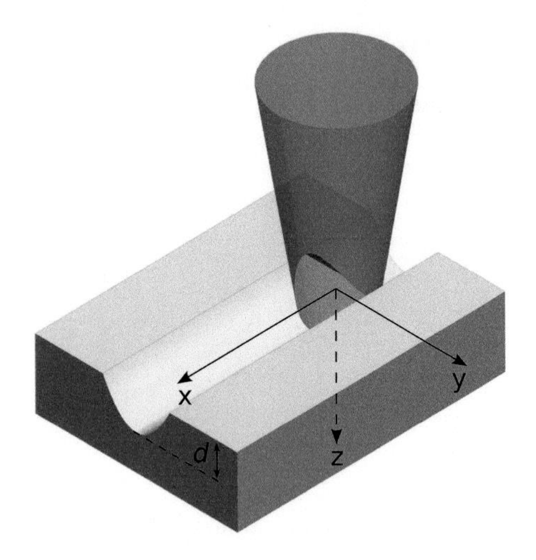

Fig. 5.1 Laser incision of soft tissue: rapid scans of the laser beam along an incision line l vaporize overlying layers of tissue with each pass. This process creates a crater on the surface of tissue, with depth d

the description of the methodology. The depth d of the incision depends on the combination of the following laser parameters: the laser power P, pulse duration τ, beam scanning frequency ω_s, plus the total laser exposure time t_{exp}. Because of the continuous nature of the output variable d, our problem is formulated in terms of a supervised regression problem: input/output data pairs are collected in order to understand and model the relation between the laser parameters and the resulting ablation depth.

Although the process we seek to model involves nonlinear physical phenomena, simple linear models exist in the literature, that provide predictions for the ablation depth based on the amount of laser energy delivered to the tissue [1].The analysis of these models provides useful directions to understand the nature of function f and, thus select an appropriate regression method for its approximation.

Prior research in the domain of laser-tissue interactions has established that the amount of material removed by thermal ablation depends primarily on the spatial distribution of energy density E [1, 2]. Estimations for the laser ablation depth can be computed by means of simple heuristic models. These are based on the assumption that material removal occurs as a continuous steady-state process, i.e. at a fixed, time-invariant rate. This assumption is legitimate if long laser pulses are used, i.e. $\tau > 1\,\mu\text{s}$ [1].

In a steady-state model, the removal of a unit mass of tissue requires the absorption of a fixed amount of energy, quantified by the *ablation enthalpy* h_{abl} ($\text{J} \cdot \text{kg}^{-1}$). Assuming a tissue with uniform density ρ, the relation between the depth of ablation d and the applied energy density E is described by [1]

$$d = \frac{E - E_{th}}{\rho \cdot h_{abl}}, \tag{5.1}$$

where E_{th} is the *ablation threshold*, i.e. the minimum amount of energy required to initiate the material removal process. Such threshold depends on the coefficient of absorption of tissue μ_a, according to the following relation

$$E_{th} = \frac{\rho \cdot h_{abl}}{\mu_a}. \tag{5.2}$$

Because of their simplicity, these models allow for a rapid, albeit rough estimation of the ablation depth. In practice, their application requires a prior determination of the ablation enthalpy h_{abl}, which is not straightforward to accomplish. Based on Eq. 5.1, this quantity can be estimated as the slope of a linear fitting between the ablation depth and the energy density,

$$h_{abl} = \frac{\Delta E}{\rho \Delta d}. \tag{5.3}$$

Nonetheless, this empirical method assumes that the energy density E emitted by the laser is entirely absorbed in the tissue: this assumption may not hold under all circumstances, since numerous factors exist that induce attenuations or alterations of the laser beam. For instance, previous studies have shown that absorption losses in the ablation plume can attenuate the laser energy up to 40 % of its theoretical value [1].

Despite the applicability issues mentioned above, steady-state models provide a basic understanding of the energetics of thermal ablation processes. These models postulate a linear relation between the ablation depth and the laser energy density E. This is surprising, especially in the light of our knowledge of the mechanisms involved in thermal ablation processes: the deposition of laser energy within tissue determines the onset of complex physical interactions, most of which are nonlinear in nature. Nonetheless, experimental studies show that under specific circumstances the relation between laser energy and ablation depth can be as simple as a linear function [3, 4], suggesting that the magnitude of nonlinear effects is neglectable.

5.2 Influencing Parameters

Our approach aims to extend the framework of steady-state models, investigating the individual contribution of each of the laser parameters. Understanding and modeling these contributions will allow for the creation of more explicit models of ablation depth, that use the same set of inputs used by clinicians during surgery, thus being straightforward to implement in a surgical context.

In this section we describe the experiments carried out to determine the influence of the energy delivery mode and the frequency of the laser scanning motion on the depth of incision produced by the laser exposure.

5.2.1 *Influence of Energy Delivery Mode*

Laser sources allow to control the rate of energy transfer by means of different *delivery modes*. In general, a delivery mode is defined by a function $m(t)$, which affects the energy density being delivered to the target according to the following equation:

$$E = \int_0^{t_{exp}} I\, m(t)\, dt. \quad (5.4)$$

An example is shown in Fig. 5.2, where the effects of two different delivery modes are contrasted: Continuous Wave (CW) and Repeated Pulse (RP). Using pulsed irradiation, the energy delivery process is slower, thus requiring additional exposure time to produce the same amount of energy density. When using the RP mode, the pulse duration (τ) needs to be configured. The laser source used in our experiments does not allow for an arbitrary value of duty cycle. Given a pulse duration, laser pulses are produced according to the following modulating function

$$m(t) = \sum_k (k)^{-1} H(t - k\tau), k \in \mathbb{N}, \quad (5.5)$$

where $H(t)$ is the Heaviside step function.

Here, the quantification of the effects of delivering the same amount of energy through different delivery modes was performed experimentally. To exclude the effects of laser motion on the resultant depth, single point incisions were performed, i.e. no scanning motion was applied to the laser beam, ($\omega_s = 0$). For these experiments, laser power was kept constant ($P = 2\,\text{W}$). We compared the effects of CW and RP ($\tau = 0.5\,\text{s}$) for increasing values of energy. The experiment involved three pairs

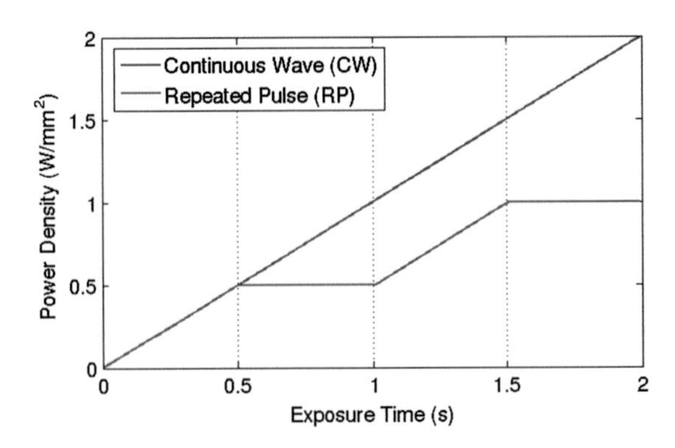

Fig. 5.2 Power densities transferred to tissue by a laser source ($I = 1\ \text{W} \cdot \text{mm}^{-2}$) by means of Continuous Wave (CW) and Repeated Pulse (RP) modes. For the RP mode, a pulse duration of 0.5 s and a duty-cycle of 50 % are considered. Reproduced from [5] with kind permission from John Wiley & Sons, Ltd

of experimental conditions. for each pair, we fixed the amount of energy involved. Experimental units were determined on the basis of actual values of energy used during real surgical interventions. Assigned values were 6, 10 and 15 joules. We performed ten repetitions for each configuration, resulting in a total of sixty ablations. Agar-based gel targets were used for this experiment.

Results

The examination of the produced ablation craters is illustrated in Fig. 5.3. Results are presented in Fig. 5.4. As expected, increasing energy densities resulted in deeper ablation craters. The experiment revealed that the ablation depth depends not just on the applied energy density, but also on the delivery mode. Under fixed energy conditions, the CW mode was found to produce, on average, deeper ablations. The difference between the mean ablation depths obtained in RP and CW was significant for values of energy equal to 10J ($p = 0.0125$) and 15J ($p = 0.0011$). In contrast, the difference was not significant at 6J ($p = 0.0823$).

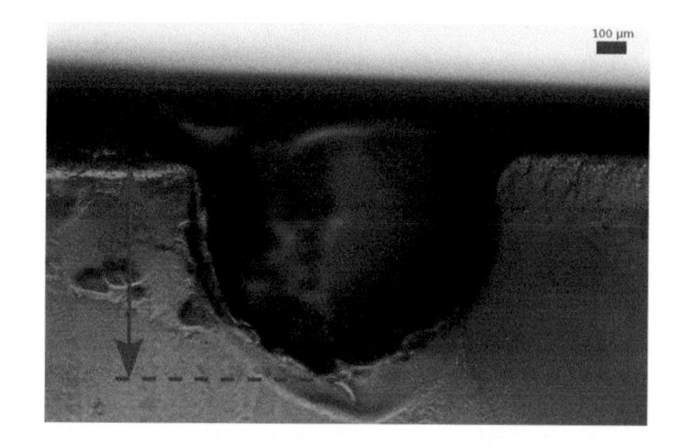

Fig. 5.3 Ablation crater produced on 2 % agar-based gel target. The resulting depth of incision *d* is indicated

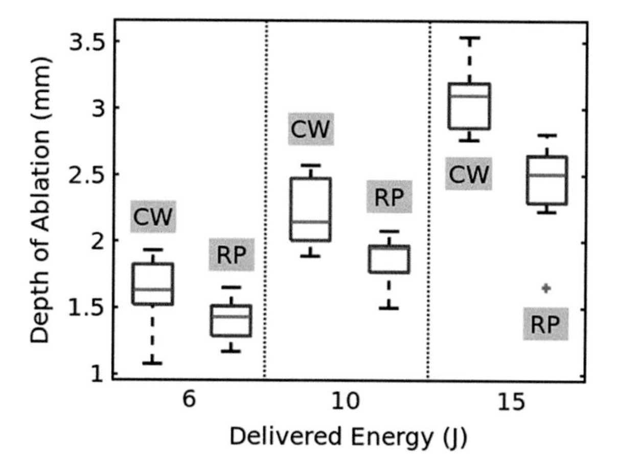

Fig. 5.4 Results of ablation depth produced with different energy delivery modes in agar-based gel targets. Reproduced from [5] with kind permission from John Wiley & Sons, Ltd

Table 5.1 Mean ($\bar{d}$), standard deviation (σ) and coefficient of variation (c_v) of ablation depths produced on agar-based gel targets through different delivery modes

Energy (J)	Delivery Mode	$\bar{d}$ (mm)	σ (mm)	c_v (%)
6	CW	1.619	0.266	16.4
	RP	1.410	0.162	11.4
10	CW	2.215	0.267	12.0
	RP	1.869	0.206	11.0
15	CW	3.075	0.254	8.2
	RP	2.421	0.356	14.7

Reproduced from [5] with kind permission from John Wiley & Sons, Ltd

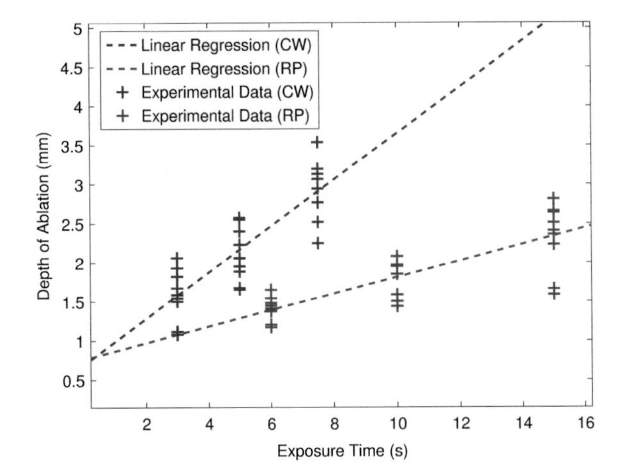

Fig. 5.5 Models of ablation depth in agar-based gel targets for Continuous Wave (*blue*) and Repeated Pulse mode (RP, *red*). Reproduced from [5] with kind permission from John Wiley & Sons, Ltd

Table 5.1 shows the average depth of incision for all the experiments; standard deviation and coefficient of variation are also listed. Observed variabilities have a marginal significance, as the coefficients of variation are all well below 20 %.

Further analysis of experimental data reveals that, once a delivery mode has been fixed, the ablation depth depends linearly on the applied exposure time. A simple linear regression is able to model the relation between these two quantities (Fig. 5.5) for both CW and RP. In both cases, the fitting error (normalized mean squared error, nMSE) is 0.02 %.

5.2.2 *Influence of Scanning Frequency*

Surgeons produce incisions by means of scans, i.e. movements of the laser beam along a trajectory on the surface of the tissue. The robotic platform used in this research [6, 7] offers automatic laser scanning, allowing for fast scans at a controlled frequency. Prior research has shown that there is a correlation between the speed of motion of the laser and the resulting depth of incision in hard tissue [4]. We wish to determine if a similar relation holds true for soft tissue. Therefore, an experiment was performed to determine the influence of the laser scanning frequency on the depth of the resulting incision.

The laser beam was fired on the flat surface of agar-based gel targets, while it was automatically scanning along a line of fixed length ($l = 4.6$ mm). The scanning frequency was controlled through the scan time (t_s), which defined the time needed to move the beam back and forth along the pre-defined scan line. Three different values of scan time were considered: 30, 50 and 100 ms. We explored the effect of these speeds at increasing values of exposure time: 3–6 s with increments of 1 s. These values of scan time and exposure time are consistent with values typically used during surgery. For each combination of scan time/exposure time, nine repeated trials were executed, resulting in a total of 108 incisions. Constant laser power (3W) and delivery mode (CW) were used throughout the entire experiment.

Results

Results are shown in Fig. 5.6. Depending on the scan time, different depths of incision were obtained. The collected data shows that there is a correlation between scan time and the depth of the resulting incision cavity. Specifically, longer scan times are observed to produce deeper incisions.

Statistics of variability for these experiments are reported in Table 5.2. With respect to the energy delivery mode experiment, results are more uniform: observed standard deviations are one order of magnitude smaller, while the coefficients of variation are all below 13 %.

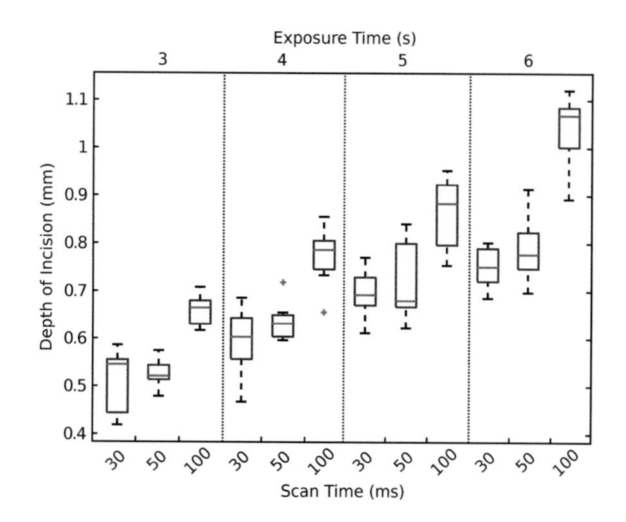

Fig. 5.6 Incision depths produced through different combinations of laser scan time/exposure time in agar-based gel targets. Reproduced from [5] with kind permission from John Wiley & Sons, Ltd

Table 5.2 Mean ($\bar{d}$), standard deviation (σ) and coefficient of variation (c_v) of ablation depths produced on agar-based gel targets through different values of scan time (t_s)

t_{exp} (s)	t_s (ms)	$\bar{d}$ (mm)	σ (mm)	c_v (%)
3	30	0.50	0.064	12.91
	50	0.63	0.037	5.9
	100	0.86	0.073	8.54
4	30	0.52	0.028	5.4
	50	0.77	0.056	7.32
	100	0.75	0.041	5.6
5	30	0.65	0.03	4.57
	50	0.69	0.045	6.69
	100	0.78	0.065	8.4
6	30	0.59	0.066	11.27
	50	0.72	0.081	11.27
	100	1.04	0.072	6.99

Reproduced from [5] with kind permission from John Wiley & Sons, Ltd

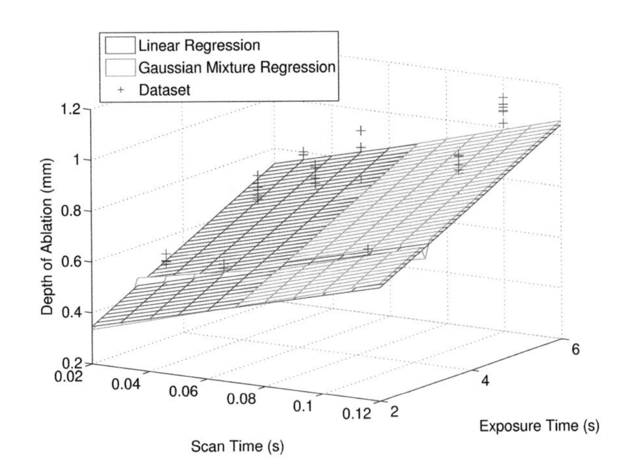

Fig. 5.7 Models of incision depth in agar-based gel targets for different combinations of scan time/exposure time. Reproduced from [5] with kind permission from John Wiley & Sons, Ltd

The combined influence of scan time and exposure time on the depth of incision is presented in Fig. 5.7. A simple linear regression of data fits the dataset with an error (normalized mean squared error, nMSE) of 0.6 %. A Gaussian mixture regression [8] was also evaluated, resulting in a fitting error of 0.8 %.

5.3 Incision Depth in Ex-Vivo Soft Tissue

During real interventions, surgeons set the laser parameters (power, delivery mode, scan time) before the execution of an incision. Exposure time is the only variable which is manipulated on-line in order to control the cutting process and the resulting incision depth. In this section, we focus on the relation between incision depth and exposure time, with the aim of modeling it. Data used to produce this model was collected during experiments involving laser incision of ex-vivo soft tissue (chicken breast).

We propose that a function f exists, mapping the laser exposure time t_{exp} to the resulting depth of incision d,

$$d = f(t_{exp}) \tag{5.6}$$

Incisions were produced to obtain representative input/output data pairs ($\{t^i_{exp}, d^i\}_{i=1,\ldots,m}$) from which the function f could be estimated.

The input range for these experiments was selected in order to include values of exposure time typically used during real laser microsurgeries. The maximum exposure time in those cases is restricted by the fact that long exposures can produce thermal damage to the tissue [9, 10]. Surgeons aim to have an exposure time that is long enough for cutting, but still sufficiently short to avoid extensive damage to the surrounding tissue. Values of exposure time were chosen randomly in the selected range (0.5 5 s). A total of 54 incision trials were performed ($P = 3W$, Continuous Wave, $t_s = 0.1$ s, $l = 4.6$ mm).

Results

Typical incision craters observed during the examination of samples are shown in Fig. 5.8. The results are shown in Fig. 5.9. It can be seen that the relation between laser exposure time and incision depth is linear in this region of the input space. Collected data was randomized and divided into a training set and a validation set of 28 and 26 data points respectively. A simple least square minimization produced a linear estimation of the training set with Root Mean Square Error (RMSE) = 0.14 mm. The estimated rate of change of the depth was 0.28 mm/s for the specific laser parameters used. The accuracy of this model was evaluated on the validation set, where an error (RMSE) of 0.10 mm was obtained.

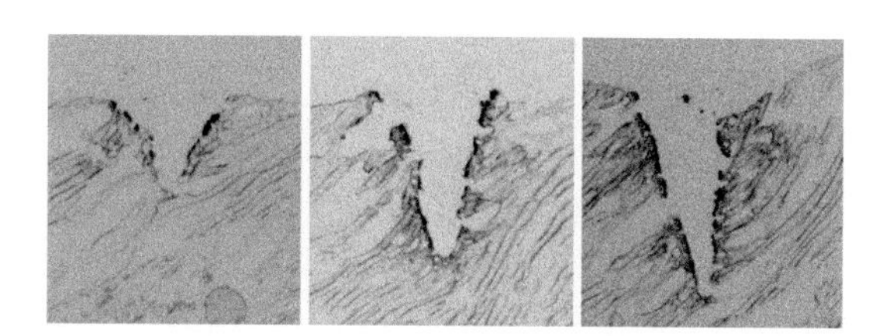

Fig. 5.8 Incision profiles produced with increasing exposure times (2.5, 3.5 and 4.5 s) and constant power density, scanning frequency and length. In order to get a complete exposure of the crater profile, targets were sectioned into thin slices (30 μm) with a cryostat microtome. Reproduced from [11]

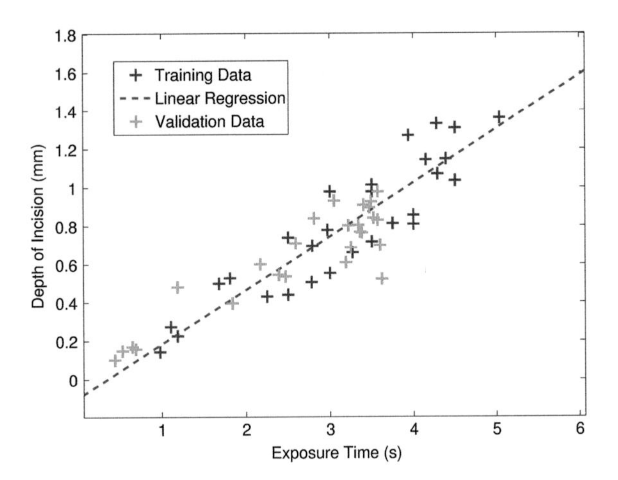

Fig. 5.9 Depth of incision in ex-vivo soft tissue for different exposure times. Reproduced from [5] with kind permission from John Wiley & Sons, Ltd

5.4 Inverse Model of Depth

Based on the linear model of depth derived in the previous section, here we create an inverse model, capable of estimating the exposure time ($\tilde{t}_{exp}$) required to achieve desired incision depths (a^*),

$$\tilde{t}_{exp} = f^{-1}(a^*). \tag{5.7}$$

This model is straightforward to obtain from the linear regression approximating Eq. 5.6. Implementing this model in the system, the exposure time is automatically controlled given a reference instead of an action.

In order to verify the quality of the estimations, five controlled experiments were conducted to estimate the prediction error. Table 5.3 shows the depths automatically obtained by the system when requiring a certain depth and using the inverse model. Discrepancies between the desired and the actual depths yield an error (RMSE) of 0.12 mm (Fig. 5.10).

Table 5.3 Results of the five automatic laser incision trials

a^* (mm)	$\tilde{t}_{exp}$ (s)	d (mm)
0.58	2.47	0.66
0.68	2.88	0.61
0.77	3.28	0.76
0.87	3.69	0.93
0.97	4.10	0.95

The desired depth $a*$ is mapped to the required exposure time $\tilde{t}_{exp}$ through an inverse model. The achieved depth d is reported in the rightmost column. Adapted from [12]

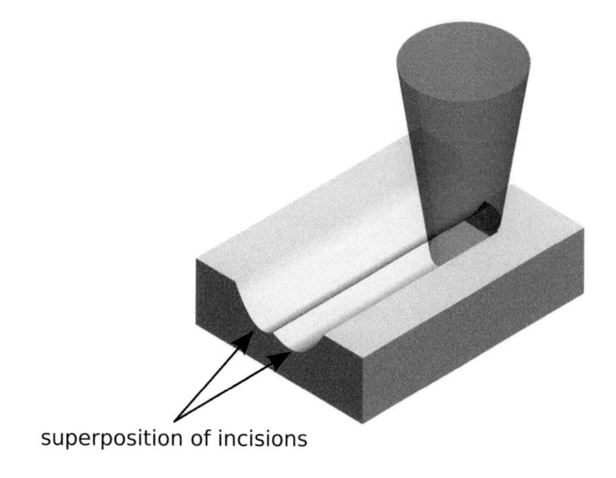

Fig. 5.10 Tissue ablation by incision superposition. Two (or more) incisions can be executed next to each other to ablate entire volumes of tissue

5.5 Ablation by Incision Superposition

Besides resecting tissue specimens and performing incisions, surgeons often require to completely eliminate blocks of tissue as part of surgical procedures. In the medical vocabulary this is known as *ablation*. This section presents a methodology to create controlled ablations based on the superposition of multiple incisions (see Fig. 5.10). The methodology uses the models of ablation depth derived in the previous section.

5.5.1 *Ablation Model*

Observing the linearity of the relationship between exposure time and incision depth, and assuming other thermal effects can be neglected (e.g., melting, carbonization) we hypothesize that the total effect of the laser exposure can be described as the sum of elemental exposures. In the case of using n incisions in parallel, the contour of the transverse plane $h(x)$ is then given by,

$$h(x) = \sum_{i}^{n} a_i \cdot \exp\left(\frac{-(x - b_i)^2}{2\sigma_i^2}\right) \tag{5.8}$$

where b_i represents the distance from the origin to the center of the ith incision. Fig. 5.11 shows an ablation generated adding four incisions. Using the model in (5.8) different strategies can be used to obtain the desired ablation depending on the required characteristics. One such strategy is described below.

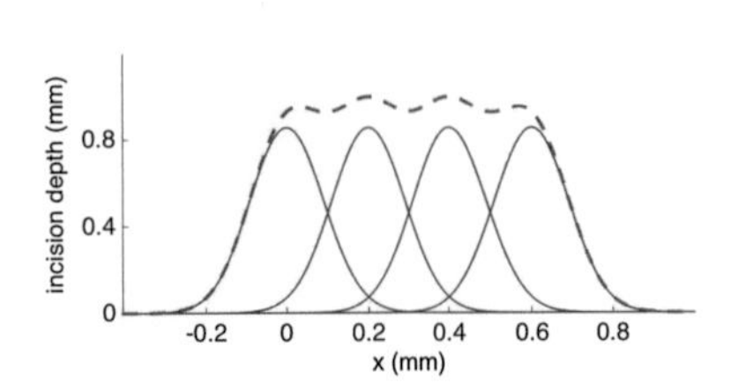

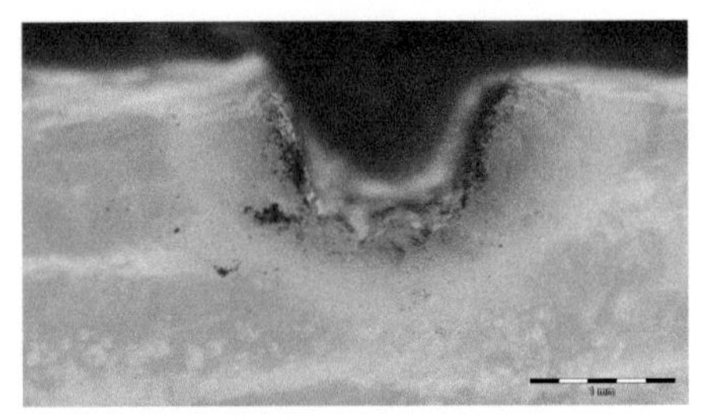

Fig. 5.11 Ablation by incision superposition. The graph on the *left* illustrates the concept: here, four incision profiles (*solid blue lines*) are combined to produce a larger ablation, whose profile is represented by the *dashed red line*. The figure on the *right* shows the transverse plane of an ablation cavity obtained by superimposing incisions on chicken muscle tissue. Adapted from [12]

5.5.2 Controlled Ablation

It can be shown that the sum of two identical Gaussians separated by a distance equal to the double of its standard deviation, i.e., $b_1 = 0, b_2 = 2\sigma$, results in a function whose maximum value is located in $(x = \sigma)$ and is given by,

$$h(\sigma) = \frac{2 \cdot a}{\sqrt{\exp(1)}} \tag{5.9}$$

Furthermore, it can be shown that the value of $h(x)$ is constant in an interval of the input space centered around $(x = \sigma)$, i.e. the function here presents a flat profile.[1]

These conditions can be used to perform a controlled ablation through the superposition of multiple incisions. A desired ablation depth (h^*) is mapped to the required incision amplitude using (5.9). The required exposure time can be obtained using the inverse model,

$$t_{exp} = f^{-1}\left(\frac{\sqrt{\exp(1)} \cdot h^*}{2}\right) \tag{5.10}$$

5.5.3 Ablation Assessment

In order to analyze the characteristics of the ablations, samples are examined under a microscope and differences among the profiles are analyzed. Repeatability of the ablation process can be studied defining a metric to compare among them. Ablation profiles are segmented, measuring the values for total width as well as depth in three different points of the crater (25, 50 and 75 % of the total width). Such metrics are described in Fig. 5.12.

[1]A proof is given in Appendix C.

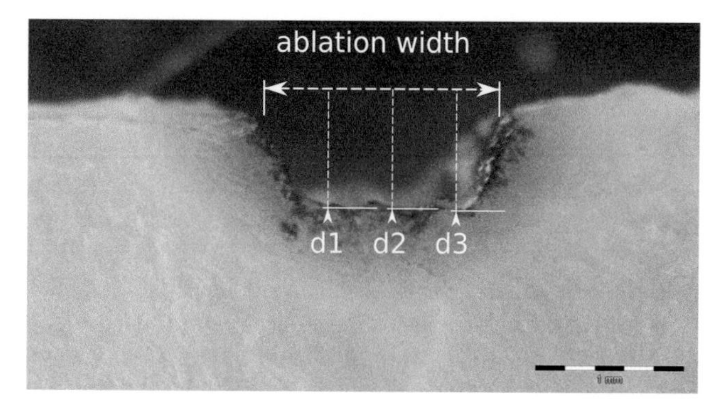

Fig. 5.12 Magnified view of an ablation profile created using the proposed automatic method. The depth of ablation is sampled in regular intervals along the ablation width. These measures are compared in order to evaluate the flatness of the ablation. Adapted from [12]

5.5.4 *Results*

Controlled Ablation

Four controlled ablations were created using the presented methodology. Given a desired ablation depth $h^* = 1.0$ mm, two incisions in parallel are required with a depth of $a^* = 0.824$ mm, which corresponds to an exposure time of $t_{exp} = 3.4$ s. Incisions must be separated a distance two times the estimated incision spread $b_2 = 2 \times \sigma$. An error (RMSE) of 0.17 mm was observed between the target depth h^* and the depths resulting from the ablations.

Ablation Assessment

The relative variability of the ablations was assessed comparing fourteen (14) ablation samples. Distribution of the observed ablation depths (d1, d2, d3) are graphically compared in Fig. 5.13. The mean ablation width was 1.62 mm.

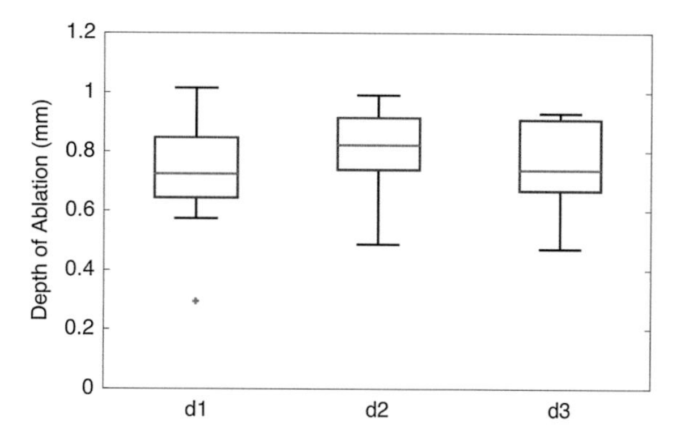

Fig. 5.13 Variability of the ablation depth at different points of the crater. The means are 0.72, 0.80 and 0.74 mm for d1, d2 and d3, respectively. Adapted from [12]

5.6 Discussion

The collected evidence shows that estimation of laser cutting depth in soft tissue can be enabled by a function that maps the laser exposure time to the resulting ablation depth. Such a function was extracted from experimental data. The described methodology allowed the creation of a model able to estimate the laser incision depth in ex-vivo chicken muscle tissue. A linear regression was found to adequately model the relation between exposure time and the laser incision depth. The model achieved a validation accuracy of 0.1 mm over incisions up to 1.4 mm deep produced on fresh ex-vivo tissue. The inverse model was used to control the laser incision depth, and to implement a strategy to perform controlled tissue ablation. The quality of the depth measurements was found to be a crucial aspect of the modeling methodology. Errors in the data can affect the function approximation task, producing inaccurate models. Although different from other methods found in the literature (e.g. confocal microscopy [13, 14]) Optical Coherence Tomography [15], Inline Coherent Imaging [16]), the protocol used in our research work presents a suitable resolution for the measurement of incision depths in the range of tenths of millimeters.

The proposed estimation method does not require any additional sensing device, thus it is appropriate for Transoral Laser Microsurgery (TLM). Considering the resection margins typically employed during TLM, we observe that the accuracy of the model is compatible with the requirements of these interventions. Surgeons aim to reach a minimum of 5 mm in resection depth to achieve surgical radicality [17, 18], i.e. to ensure the removal of the whole tumor. Smaller margins, down to 1 mm, are used in those cases where function preservation is considered, including the treatment of glottic cancer [17, 18]. However, it is important to point out that the reported accuracy was obtained on muscle tissue. Although it was used in the development of the proof-of-concept system, this type of tissue is not representative of the variety of tissues that are encountered during TLM, e.g. epithelium, muscle, adipose and fibrous tissues. These tissues present different optical properties [19], resulting in different laser absorption characteristics. This may mean that the ablation rate (mm/s) of these tissues differ from the linear relation that we have reported in this study for muscle tissue. The implementation of on-line estimation of incision depth in a real-case TLM scenario requires the availability of models able to account for the behavior of different types of tissues. Based on these observations, further experimental work might be required to study the ablation rate of different tissues and to find appropriate regression models.

All laser trials reported here present some degree of variability in the results, which can negatively affect the accuracy of the on-line depth estimation. This phenomenon has been observed in similar studies [4, 13, 14] and can be attributed to different factors. For example, instabilities of the laser source may affect the output power of the beam, producing deviations from intended values. Another limiting factor is represented by the inhomogeneous composition of biological tissue. These alterations influence the thermal interaction between laser radiation and tissue, thereby hindering the repeatability of laser incisions. However, the levels of variability observed in this study were sufficiently small not to affect the reliability of the depth estimation. Errors observed during the ex-vivo incision trials support the conclusion that the model provides reliable estimations despite the mentioned repeatability issues.

References

1. A. Vogel, V. Venugopalan, Mechanisms of pulsed laser ablation of biological tissues. Chem. Rev. **103**(2), 577–644 (2003)
2. M. Niemz, *Laser-tissue Interactions* (Springer, Berlin, 2004)
3. K. Nahen, A. Vogel, Plume dynamics and shielding by the ablation plume during er:yag laser ablation. J. Biomed. Opt. **7**(2), 165–178 (2002)
4. S. Stopp, D. Svejdar, E. von Kienlin, H. Deppe, T.C. Lueth, A new approach for creating defined geometries by navigated laser ablation based on volumetric 3-d data. IEEE Trans. Biomed. Eng. 1872–1880 (2008)
5. L. Fichera, D. Pardo, P. Illiano, J. Ortiz, D.G. Caldwell, L.S. Mattos, Online estimation of laser incision depth for transoral microsurgery: approach and preliminary evaluation. Int. J. Med. Robot. Comput. Assist. Surg. (2015). http://dx.doi.org/10.1002/rcs.1656
6. L.S. Mattos, N. Deshpande, G. Barresi, L. Guastini, G. Peretti, A novel computerized surgeon machine interface for robot-assisted laser phonomicrosurgery. Laryngoscope **124**(8), 1887–1894 (2014)
7. L. Mattos, G. Dagnino, G. Becattini, M. Dellepiane, D. Caldwell, A virtual scalpel system for computer-assisted laser microsurgery. IEEE/RSJ Int. Conf. Intell. Robots Syst. (IROS) **2011**, 1359–1365 (2011)
8. S. Calinon, Robot Programming by Demonstration: A Probabilistic Approach (EPFL/CRC Press, 2009)
9. D. Pardo, L. Fichera, D. Caldwell, L. Mattos, Learning temperature dynamics on agar-based phantom tissue surface during single point co_2 laser exposure. Neural Process. Lett. **42**(1), 55–70 (2015). http://dx.doi.org/10.1007/s11063-014-9389-y
10. L. Fichera, D. Pardo, and L. S. Mattos, in *Supervisory System for Robot Assisted Laser Phonomicrosurgery*. Proceedings of the 35th International Conference of the IEEE Engineering in Medicine and Biology Society (EMBC), 2013
11. L. Fichera, D. Pardo, D.G. Caldwell, L.S. Mattos, in *New Assistive Technologies for Laser Microsurgery*. 4th Joint Workshop on New Technologies for Computer/Robot Assisted Surgery (CRAS-2014) (2014), pp. 60–63
12. L. Fichera, D. Pardo, P. Illiano, D. Caldwell, L. Mattos, in *Feed Forward Incision Control for Laser Microsurgery of Soft Tissue*. 2015 IEEE International Conference on Robotics and Automation (ICRA) (2015), pp. 1235–1240

13. L.A. Kahrs, J. Burgner, T. Klenzner, J. Raczkowsky, J. Schipper, H. Wörn, Planning and simulation of microsurgical laser bone ablation. Int. J. Comput. Assist. Radiol. Surg. **5**(2), 155–162 (2010)
14. J. Burgner, M. Müller, J. Raczkowsky, H. Wörn, Ex vivo accuracy evaluation for robot assisted laser bone ablation. Int. J. Med. Robot. Comput. Assist. Surg. **6**(4), 489–500 (2010)
15. H.W. Kang, J. Oh, A.J. Welch, Investigations on laser hard tissue ablation under various environments. Phys. Med. Biol. **53**(12), 3381 (2008)
16. B.Y. Leung, P.J. Webster, J.M. Fraser, V.X. Yang, Real-time guidance of thermal and ultrashort pulsed laser ablation in hard tissue using inline coherent imaging. Lasers Surg. Med. **44**(3), 249–256 (2012)
17. M.L. Hinni, A. Ferlito, M.S. Brandwein-Gensler, R.P. Takes, C.E. Silver, W.H. Westra, R.R. Seethala, J.P. Rodrigo, J. Corry, C.R. Bradford, J.L. Hunt, P. Strojan, K.O. Devaney, D.R. Gnepp, D.M. Hartl, L.P. Kowalski, A. Rinaldo, L. Barnes, Surgical margins in head and neck cancer: A contemporary review. Head Neck **35**(9), 1362–1370 (2013)
18. G. Mannelli, G. Meccariello, A. Deganello, V. Maio, D. Massi, O. Gallo, Impact of low-thermal-injury devices on margin ststus in laryngeal cancer. an experiment ex vivo study. Oral Oncol. **50**(1), 32–39 (2014)
19. S.L. Jacques, Optical properties of biological tissues: a review. Phys. Med. Biol. **58**(11), R37 (2013)

Chapter 6
Realization of a Cognitive Supervisory System for Laser Microsurgery

Based on the models presented in Chaps. 4 and 5, here we describe the development of a prototypical supervisory system for laser microsurgery. The objective is to prove the concept formulated in Chap. 3 of a system capable of monitoring (i) the superficial temperature of tissues and (ii) the laser cutting depth during a surgical intervention.

As mentioned in the introduction of this dissertation, the work presented here is part of a broader research effort carried out at the Istituto Italiano di Tecnologia (IIT), in the scope of the European project μRALP. This research recently culminated in the development of a novel computer-assisted surgical platform for laryngeal laser procedures, called the "μRALP Surgical System". The Cognitive Supervisor is implemented as a software component and integrated to this platform.

This chapter begins with a description of the μRALP Surgical System and the hardware components it involves. Then, a technical description of the Cognitive Supervisory System is given, with a focus on its integration within the μRALP System. Finally, we report on a preliminary evaluation study, aiming to verify the system's performance in an operational context. Laser trials were performed, in which users' performance in tasks involving incisions to a pre-specified depth were assessed.

6.1 Introduction: The μRALP Surgical System

The μRALP System is an experimental surgical system for laryngeal laser procedures. The system's concept is illustrated in Fig. 6.1: this is inspired by the setup currently in use for transoral laser microsurgeries (TLM) (which was described in Sect. 3.1). The μRALP system represents a revised, computer-assisted version of traditional TLM systems.

In the following, we give a description of the hardware and software components of the system.

L. Fichera, *Cognitive Supervision for Robot-Assisted Minimally Invasive Laser Surgery*, Springer Theses, DOI 10.1007/978-3-319-30330-7_6

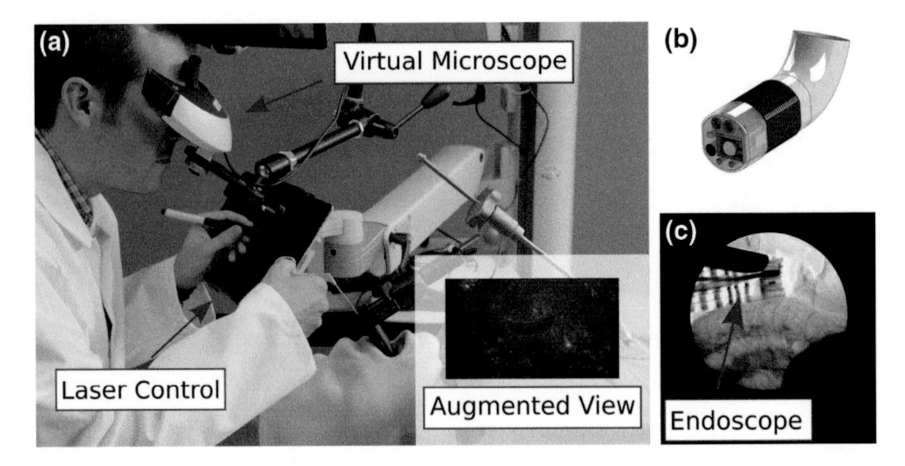

Fig. 6.1 The μRALP system concept. Here, the surgeon visualizes the surgical site through a *virtual microscope* device based on modified head-mounted display (HMD). These device is amenable to the display of virtual overlays that can be used to graphically display additional information, e.g. an intraoperative ablation plan. The position of the laser beam is controlled with a commercial input device (stylus and graphics tablet). An endoscopic device (**b**) brings the laser beam in proximity of the surgical site [1] (image courtesy of Dennis Kundrat, Leibniz Universität Hannover). The endoscope is equipped with a microscopic mirror that enables laser motion. The X-Ray image in (**c**) shows the insertion of the endoscope in the larynx (sagittal plane).

6.1.1 Hardware Components

The μRALP system comprises the following components:

Flexible Endoscope

This device, whose first prototype is described in [1], is inserted in the larynx of the patient; it delivers the laser to the surgical field through an internal laser fiber. An actuated micro-mirror on the distal tip provides the means for laser motion [2]. Visualization of the surgical field is enabled by a pair of miniaturized high-definition cameras mounted on tip.

Surgeon Console

The console comprises a laser control device (a WACOM Bamboo Pen and Touch graphics tablet) and a *virtual microscope*, i.e. a stereoscopic head-mount display (SONY HMZ-T2 - 720p) that presents the stereoscopic video stream produced by the endoscope [3]. The commands imparted by the surgeon are mapped into corresponding laser beam trajectories on the surgical site. Motion scaling allows clinicians to work at a convenient scale, while their actions are adapted to the minuscule size of the target.

The console offers two distinct operating modes, called *virtual scalpel* and *intra-operative planning*. The former allows real-time user control of both laser aiming and activation; the latter modality enables the planning of laser incision/ablation patterns that, once approved, are automatically executed by the system. Plans are defined and previewed in the virtual microscope, through the superimposition of virtual overlays. Both operating modes are supplemented with the possibility to define safety region overlays, i.e. regions within the surgical area where the laser is either (i) allowed to operate or (ii) automatically inhibited, e.g. because it contains delicate structures that must be preserved.

Configuration Interface

This is an external display that provides supplementary visualization of the surgical field for other members of the surgical team. Through this device, an assistant can perform tasks such as system configuration or selection of the operating mode.

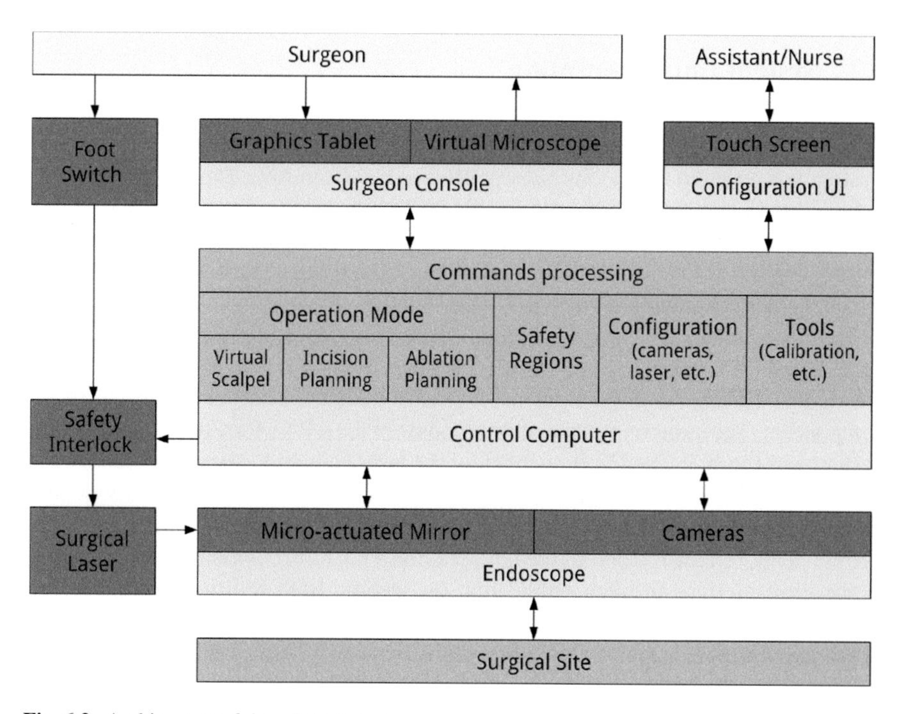

Fig. 6.2 Architecture of the μRALP System

Control Computer

A control computer coordinates the interaction among all the components of the system, as the schematic depiction in Fig. 6.2 shows. The computer is in charge of processing user commands and verify their execution. If a hardware fault is detected, the computer may disable the laser output through a safety interlock, thus preventing potential patient injury.

6.1.2 Software Architecture

The μRALP system adopts a distributed software architecture: different components are managed by distinct software modules, each instantiated as a separate Operating System process. These processes interact through a message passing scheme, with the Robot Operating System (ROS) [4] being used as communication middleware. The inclusion of a new module in the system requires the specification of its interface, i.e. the information it exchanges with other processed of the system.

6.2 System Implementation

This section describes the realization and integration of the Cognitive Supervisory System within the μRALP Surgical platform. The Cognitive Supervisory System is intended to complement the clinician's perception of the state of tissues during the laser incision process, through the visualization of estimated values of the laser cutting depth and the superficial temperature of the tissue. The estimations rely on the mathematical models derived in Chaps. 4 and 5.

Here, the models are encapsulated into shared libraries and instantiated by a ROS node called the Cognitive Supervisor (CS). This module is responsible for feeding the models with the required input and for distributing their output to other software components. The interconnection of this module in the μRALP software architecture is shown in Fig. 6.3. The CS is enabled by the laser activation signal emitted by the laser controller (ROS Actionlib). During the application of laser power on tissue, the supervisor module produces two distinct messages; these contain estimations of the current depth of incision and tissue temperature. This information is made available to the user interface through publication on specific ROS topics. To produce the estimations mentioned above, the CS needs to know the laser dosimetry parameters in use (laser power, scanning frequency, delivery mode). These parameters are set by an assistant through the configuration interface and made available under the form of ROS parameters.

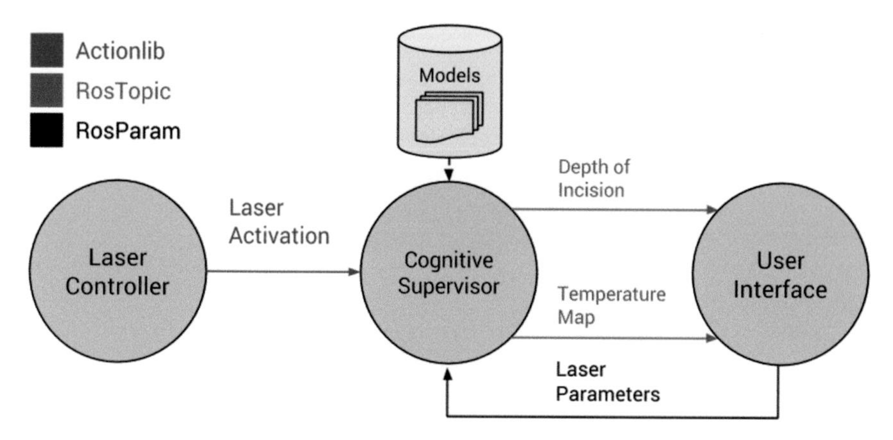

Fig. 6.3 Coordination of the software processes involved in the on-line estimation of laser cutting depth/thermal state of tissue. The estimations are calculated by the Cognitive Supervisor (CS), based on mathematical models that are loaded from file. The laser parameters required to calculate the estimations are received from the User Interface. The CS is synchronized with the activation signal produced by the Laser Controller. When the laser is activated, the CS delivers the output of the models to the User Interface, by means of a continuous flow of messages

6.2.1 Software Architecture

The class diagram of Fig. 6.4 illustrates the software architecture on which the Cognitive Supervisor is based. An `App` class encapsulates the data structures required by the module: this includes instances of the ROS publishers and subscribers required to establish connections with other ROS nodes in system.

The Cognitive Supervisor implements a simple finite state machine with two states, namely `Idle` and `LaserOn`. This is modeled in the software architecture through the implementation of a *State* design pattern [5]. State transitions are handled in the main application loop, on the basis of the laser activation signal, which is polled at a frequency of 100 Hz.

The `PublishInfo()` method is routinely called in the main loop of the application. Exploiting the *dynamic polymorphism* offered by C++, this method performs different operations, according to the state of the application. The `Idle` class implements a *null* behavior [5]. By contrast, the `LaserOn` class performs the following sequence of operations:

1. estimation of the superficial temperature of tissue
2. estimation of the laser cutting depth
3. publishing the above information to the user interface

In its attributes, the `LaserOn` class stores the values of the laser parameters in use (laser power, scanning frequency, delivery mode). Estimations of temperature and cutting depth are demanded to classes defined in separate libraries (`DepthModel` and `TemperatureModel`).

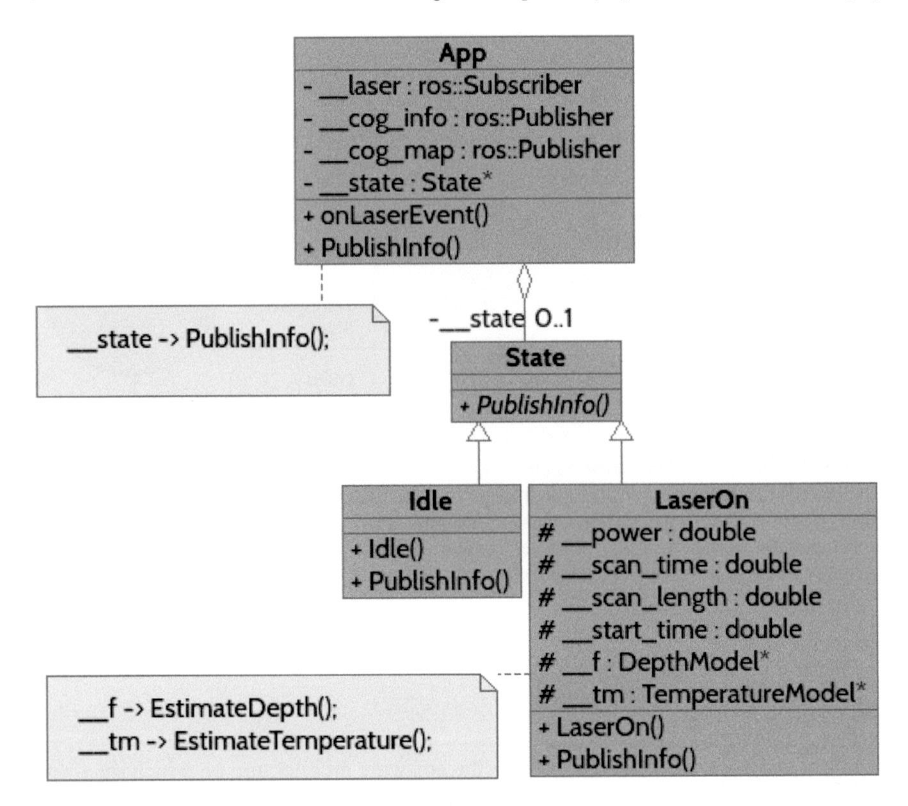

Fig. 6.4 Class diagram of Cognitive Supervisor module

When in the `LaserOn` state, the CS publishes messages containing the current estimation for the depth of incision and the superficial temperature of tissues. The specification of these messages—in the ROS message description language—is reported in Listings 6.1 and 6.2.

Listing 6.1 Definition of `cog_info` message

```
# header of the ROS msg (timestamp, etc.)
Header  header

# current depth of incision
float32 depth
```

Listing 6.2 Definition of `cog_map` message

```
# header of the ROS msg (timestamp, etc.)
Header                header

# superficial temperature of tissue
```

```
sensor_msgs/Image temp

# transformation and visualization parameters
float32          left
float32          top
float32          width
float32          height
float32          opacity
```

The `cog_map` message contains a `temp` attribute: this is a two-dimensional matrix (size: 40×60 elements) representing the superficial temperature of tissue in the surroundings of the incision. Additional attributes are provided with the message: these provide a spatial mapping between the temperature surface estimated by the cognitive supervisor and the camera view of the μRALP system. The purpose of these attributes is to provide the user interface with the information required to correctly overlap the temperature surface with the images of the surgical site.

6.2.2 Integration with the Surgical Console

The surgeon console was customized to display the information produced by the CS (see Fig. 6.5). Two widgets (graphical control elements) were added to the surgical viewer, which show (i) the superficial temperature of tissues and (ii) the progression

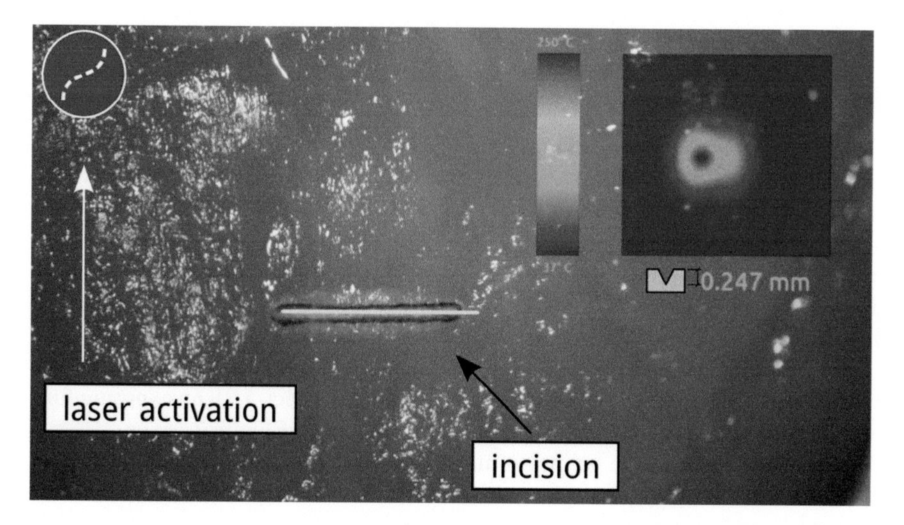

Fig. 6.5 On-line monitoring of tissue temperature and laser cutting depth. A number indicates the depth of incision in millimeters. The superficial temperature of tissue is represented through a color map which is superimposed on the surgical visor. The laser activation indicator, on the *left*, turns red if the laser is on

of the incision depth. The former is represented by a colored overlay (heat map), while the latter is indicated numerically (in millimeters). These widgets can be enabled/disabled by the assistant through the configuration interface.

6.3 Towards Assistive Technologies for Laser Microsurgery

The implementation of the Cognitive Supervisory System described in this chapter provides the groundwork for further research in the domain of computer-assisted laser surgery. The system is capable of providing useful information regarding the state of tissues during laser surgery. This enables the creation of assistive technologies potentially resulting in safer and more accurate laser resections.

Here, we present a proof-of-concept study, that exploits the depth estimation capabilities of the CS to guide users during laser cutting. Tree volunteers were involved in this study. They were all members of the scientific staff at the Istituto Italiano di Tecnologia, and had limited or no prior experience with laser incision of soft tissue. Participants were asked to perform a simple task involving control of the laser exposure time to create a specific depth of incision ($d^* = 0.85$ mm). The incision path was pre-programmed through software and kept constant throughout the experiment. Laser parameters were configured as follows: $P = 3$W, Continuous Wave, $t_s = 0.1$s, $\omega_s = 10$Hz, $l = 4.6$mm.

Each participant performed a total of six trials. In the first three trials they were required to accomplish the task only relying on their visual perception. During the three subsequent trials, they were supported with on-line estimation of depth.

Results

A comparison of the incision depths produced with and without the support of the on-line estimation system is shown in Fig. 6.6a. None of the users obtained incisions closer than 0.25 mm to the assigned target depth (0.85 mm) during the non-assisted trials. Conversely, with the support of the on-line estimation system, users produced incisions much closer to the assigned target. Deviations from the target depth are summarized in Table 6.1.

The exposure times employed by users for each of these trials are represented in Fig. 6.6b. According to the forward model of depth (see Sect. 5.3), an exposure time of $t_{exp} = 3.36$ s is required to cut a depth of 0.85 mm. From the figure it can be observed that, with the support of the online estimation system, users produced exposure times close to this reference value. Mean deviations from the target exposure time were 0.12, 0.04 and 0.10 s for each user, respectively.

At the present time, no other real-time assistive system exists to monitor and inform surgeons about the effects of the laser on tissues during the execution of incisions. Results of these trials suggest that on-line estimation of depth is beneficial to

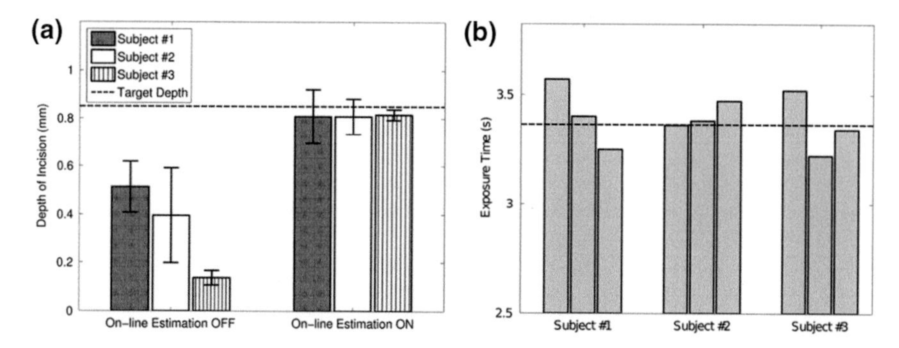

Fig. 6.6 Results of user trials. The plot on the *left* (**a**) shows the user control of incision depth with and without the support of the on-line estimation system. Measures of spread (standard deviation) are graphically represented for each sequence of trials. (**b**) shows the user control of exposure time during assisted trials (on-line estimation of depth was enabled during these trials). The target exposure time (3.36 s) is plotted for reference. Reproduced from [6] with kind permission from John Wiley & Sons, Ltd

Table 6.1 Deviations (RMSE) from the assigned incision depth obtained by users with and without the assistance of the on-line depth estimation

	Unassisted	Assisted
User 1	0.34	0.10
User 2	0.48	0.07
User 3	0.71	0.03

Figures are in millimeters. Reproduced from [6] with kind permission from John Wiley & Sons, Ltd

users who have no prior experience with laser operations. Providing depth estimations during the execution of laser incisions enabled inexperienced users to perform precise tissue cutting.

References

1. D. Kundrat, A. Schoob, B. Munske, T. Ortmaier, Towards an endoscopic device for laser-assisted phonomicrosurgery, in *Proceedings of the Hamlyn Symposium on Medical Robotics* (2013)
2. S. Lescano, D. Zlatanov, M. Rakotondrabe, N. Andreff, Kinematic analysis of a meso-scale parallel robot for laser phonomicrosurgery, ed. by A. Kecskemèthy, F. Geu Flores, in *Interdisciplinary Applications of Kinematics*. Mechanisms and Machine Science, vol. 26 (Springer International Publishing, 2015), pp. 127–135
3. N. Deshpande, J. Ortiz, D. Caldwell, L. Mattos, Enhanced computer-assisted laser microsurgeries with a "virtual microscope" based surgical system, in *2014 IEEE International Conference on Robotics and Automation (ICRA)*, May 2014, pp. 4194–4199
4. M. Quigley, K. Conley, B.P. Gerkey, J. Faust, T. Foote, J. Leibs, R. Wheeler, A.Y. Ng, Ros: an open-source robot operating system, in *ICRA Workshop on Open Source Software* (2009)
5. E. Gamma, R. Helm, R. Johnson, J. Vlissides, Design Patterns: Elements of Reusable Object-Oriented Software (Pearson Education, London, 1994)
6. L. Fichera, D. Pardo, P. Illiano, J. Ortiz, D. G. Caldwell, L.S. Mattos, Online estimation of laser incision depth for transoral microsurgery: approach and preliminary evaluation. Int. J. Med. Robot. Comput. Assist. Surg. (2015). http://dx.doi.org/10.1002/rcs.1656 (Online)

Chapter 7
Conclusions and Future Research Directions

This chapter presents a conclusion to the work described in this doctoral dissertation. The main contributions are summarized, followed by some suggestions regarding future directions of research related to this work.

7.1 Concluding Remarks

The main thrust of this thesis is to enable the automatic monitoring of laser-induced changes on tissues during robot-assisted laser microsurgery. Two types of effects were studied: thermal (tissue temperature variation) and mechanical (creation of the incision crater). Surgeon control of these effects is crucial to surgical outcomes, yet these are difficult to perceive and require a significant amount of cognitive acuity. Computer and robot-assisted surgical systems should extend the surgeon performance beyond the limitations of human possibilities, not just in terms of what the surgeon is able to do, but also in the perception of relevant processes that are difficult or impossible to sense. Drawing on these practical problems, this doctoral dissertation focused on the development of models capable of describing the changes induced by surgical lasers on soft tissues, under the condition that these models must be compatible with use in a real surgical setting.

This dissertation successfully demonstrates the applicability of statistical learning methods to model the laser incision process during laser microsurgery. To the best of our knowledge, it is the first time that these techniques are applied in this field: analytical models constitute the traditional approach for the analysis of the interaction of the laser with the tissue [1]. With respect to existing approaches, our modeling methodology explicitly considers typical laser parameters used by clinicians during an intervention, (i.e. power, scanning frequency, energy delivery mode, incision length and laser exposure time), thus producing models that are straightforward to use in a surgical scenario either for monitoring or control applications.

L. Fichera, *Cognitive Supervision for Robot-Assisted Minimally Invasive Laser Surgery*, Springer Theses, DOI 10.1007/978-3-319-30330-7_7

The key findings and novel contributions of this doctoral research are summarized below.

1. Definition of an approach to learn the superficial temperature of tissues during laser incision. The Gaussian temperature profile induced by a single TEM_{00} laser pulse is used as a basis function to represent the evolution of temperature in the area surrounding the ablation site (Sect. 4.2). The temperature variation induced by a scanning laser beam is modeled through the superposition of Gaussian functions (Sect. 4.3), achieving an average estimation error (Root-Mean-Square Error, RMSE) of 1.52 °C, and a maximum error of 2.62 °C.
2. Definition of an approach to learn the laser incision depth in soft tissues. Our approach extends existing empirical models by taking into account the individual effect of each laser parameter on the resulting incision depth (Sect. 5.2). The depth is modeled as a function of the laser exposure time. The approach was validated on ex-vivo chicken muscle tissue: it was found that a simple linear regression provides an adequate approximation of the relationship exposure time and the resulting incision depth (Sect. 5.3). Experimental validation reveals a RMSE of 0.10 mm, for incisions up to 1 mm in depth.
3. This dissertation explored the automatic control of the laser incision depth, based on a learned model that maps a desired incision depth to the laser exposure time required for its realization (Sect. 5.5). The achieved accuracy is (RMSE) 0.12 mm. In addition, we provided a novel strategy to implement the automatic ablation of entire volumes of tissue, based on the superposition of controlled laser incisions. This approach allows for the creation of ablations with pre-defined depth, with an accuracy (RMSE) of 0.17 mm.
4. A Cognitive Supervisory System (CS) prototype was developed and integrated in the μRALP surgical system. Based on the aforementioned models of temperature and incision depth, the CS endows the μRALP system with new functionalities that provide surgeons with additional information regarding the state of tissues during the execution of laser incision (Sect. 6.2):
    - The depth estimation is meant to guide the surgeon in the execution of precise tissue incisions.
    - The temperature estimation is intended to support his decisions in order to avoid thermal damage (e.g. carbonization).

7.2 Future Research Directions

The contributions in this dissertation can lead to new lines of inquiry in the area of robot-assisted laser surgery. Several new questions emerge in light of the discoveries presented here. A few of the most prominent are listed here.

7.2.1 Clinical Translation

Ex-vivo chicken muscle tissue was used to develop and validate the modeling approaches described in Chaps. 4 and 5. Translation of the presented research to clinical technologies requires one additional validation step, which is the creation of models capable of describing laser-induced changes in diverse human tissues (e.g. dermis, ligament). In-vitro models [2] seem a promising option for an initial validation: these are created by means of tissue engineering techniques that allow to replicate the composition and properties of real tissues.

7.2.2 Online Learning

A natural extension of the modeling methodologies proposed in this dissertation would be to explore on-line learning algorithms to build models that can be continuously improved, through the addition of new experimental data.

7.2.3 Automatic Control of Tissue Thermal Damage

The model of tissue temperature presented in Chap. 4 was implemented in the μRALP system. Activation and deactivation of the model is synchronized by the system, allowing online estimation of the temperature of the tissue surface. This thermal monitoring can be used to define policies to prevent thermal damage on the tissue. For instance, modification of the scanning frequency or deactivation of the laser exposure can be manipulated by the central system based on the output of the model.

7.2.4 Training of Laser Surgeons

Evidence presented in Sect. 6.3 seem to indicate that a numerical representation of the laser incision depth might help people with no prior experience of laser operations in conducting precise incisions. It would be interesting to investigate whether this could be exploited to support the training of prospective laser surgeons, specifically with respect to the the development of their laser cutting technique.

References

1. M. Niemz, *Laser-tissue Interactions* (Springer, Berlin, 2004)
2. F. Urciuolo, G. Imparato, A. Totaro, P.A. Netti, Building a tissue in vitro from the bottom up: implications in regenerative medicine. Methodist DeBakey Cardiovasc. J. **9**(4), 213 (2013)

Appendix A
Requirements Questionnaire

Given a surgical system dedicated to laser surgery of the larynx, please rate the features proposed below using the following [0–6] scale:

[0] The feature is not desirable at all

[1–5] This is a relevant feature (How much?)

[6] This feature is imperative

1. The system is able to perform **incision lines** (scanning the beam from 0.4 to 5.0 mm)
2. The system is able to perform **long incision lines** (scanning the beam from 1.0 to 2.0 cm)
3. The system is able to perform circular **ablation areas** (radius from 0.4 to 4.0 mm)
4. The system is able to perform **large ablation areas** (radius from 0.5 to 10 mm)
5. The surgeon is able to define a desired **incision depth** (from 0.4 to 2.0 mm with 0.4 mm resolution)
6. The resolution of the **depth** is 0.2 (rather than 0.4 mm)
7. The surgeon has continuous information about the approximate **temperature** of tissue during incision
8. The surgeon has continuous information about the **probability of tissue carbonization** during incision (Visual Feedback: 0–100 %)
9. The system has the possibility to **automatically decrease the power** of the laser when detecting the possibility of carbonization in a given area

L. Fichera, *Cognitive Supervision for Robot-Assisted Minimally Invasive Laser Surgery*, Springer Theses, DOI 10.1007/978-3-319-30330-7

Appendix B
Solution to the Homogeneous Heat Conduction Equation

The homogeneous heat conduction equation (Eq. 4.5) describes the temporal evolution of tissue temperature after laser exposure. Assuming a Cartesian reference frame (x, y, z), here we show that this equation has a general solution of the form

$$T(x, y, z, t) = T_0 + \frac{\alpha}{(4\pi \kappa t)^{\frac{3}{2}}} \exp\left(-\frac{x^2 + y^2 + z^2}{4\kappa t}\right), \tag{B.1}$$

where α is an integration constant. The proof is largely based on [1]: we simply assume that the temperature function defined above is a valid solution to Eq. 4.5. If this assumption is true, then replacing all occurrences of T in Eq. 4.5 will produce an identity.

As a preliminary step, let us define the term $T - T_0$: based on Eq. 4.5 we can write:

$$T - T_0 = \frac{\alpha}{(4\pi \kappa t)^{\frac{3}{2}}} \exp\left(-\frac{x^2 + y^2 + z^2}{4\kappa t}\right). \tag{B.2}$$

We first work on the left hand side of Eq. 4.5, deriving the temperature function T with respect to time. This yields the following relation:

$$\dot{T} = \frac{(6\kappa t - x^2 - y^2 - z^2) \exp\left(-\frac{x^2+y^2+z^2}{4\kappa t}\right)}{32\, \pi^{\frac{3}{2}}\, \kappa^{\frac{5}{2}}\, t^{\frac{7}{2}}}, \tag{B.3}$$

which can be rewritten in the following compact form:

$$\dot{T} = -\frac{3}{2} \frac{(T - T_0)}{2\, t} + \frac{x^2 + y^2 + z^2}{4\, \kappa\, t} (T - T_0). \tag{B.4}$$

The Laplace operator on the right hand side of Eq. 4.5 contains second-order derivatives of the temperature function T with respect to each of the Cartesian axis (x, y, z). Therefore, we shall write:

L. Fichera, *Cognitive Supervision for Robot-Assisted Minimally Invasive Laser Surgery*, Springer Theses, DOI 10.1007/978-3-319-30330-7

$$\frac{\partial^2}{\partial x^2}T = \frac{x^2(T - T_0)}{4(\kappa t)^2} - \frac{T - T_0}{2\kappa t}, \tag{B.5}$$

$$\frac{\partial^2}{\partial y^2}T = \frac{y^2(T - T_0)}{4(\kappa t)^2} - \frac{T - T_0}{2\kappa t}, \tag{B.6}$$

$$\frac{\partial^2}{\partial z^2}T = \frac{z^2(T - T_0)}{4(\kappa t)^2} - \frac{T - T_0}{2\kappa t}. \tag{B.7}$$

Based on these results, Eq. 4.5 can be rewritten as:

$$\begin{aligned}&-\frac{3}{2}\frac{(T - T_0)}{2t} + \frac{x^2 + y^2 + z^2}{4\kappa t}(T - T_0)\\ &= \kappa\left(\frac{x^2(T - T_0)}{4(\kappa t)^2} + \frac{y^2(T - T_0)}{4(\kappa t)^2} + \frac{z^2(T - T_0)}{4(\kappa t)^2} - 3\frac{T - T_0}{2\kappa t}\right).\end{aligned} \tag{B.8}$$

From some straightforward simplifications, it follows that:

$$-\frac{3}{2}\frac{(T - T_0)}{2t} + \frac{x^2 + y^2 + z^2}{4\kappa t}(T - T_0) = (T - T_0)\frac{x^2 + y^2 + z^2}{4\kappa t^2} - \frac{3}{2}\frac{(T - T_0)}{2t} \quad \blacksquare \tag{B.9}$$

Reference

1. M. Niemz, *Laser-tissue Interactions*. Springer Berlin Heidelberg, 2004.

Appendix C
Gaussian Ablation Shape

Let us define a function g as the sum of n Gaussian functions, i.e.

$$g(x) = \sum_{i}^{n} f_i(x) \tag{C.1}$$

where,

$$f_i(x) = a_i \cdot \exp\left[\frac{(x-\mu_i)^2}{2\sigma_i^2}\right]. \tag{C.2}$$

Here we assume that $\sigma_i = \sigma$, $a_i = a\ \forall i$.

We wish to find the sequence of μ_i, $i = 1, \ldots, n$ for which the resulting g function has a *top hat* flat profile, as illustrated in Fig. C.1. For the sake of simplicity, here we consider the problem for the case of two Gaussians, i.e. $n = 2$. The proof described below can be easily generalized for $n > 2$.

Let us assume that the first Gaussian is centered at the origin ($\mu_1 = 0$), then the expanded summation in Eq. C.1 is given by:

$$g(x) = a \cdot \exp\left[-\frac{x^2}{2\sigma^2}\right] + a \cdot \exp\left[-\frac{(x-\mu)^2}{2\sigma^2}\right]. \tag{C.3}$$

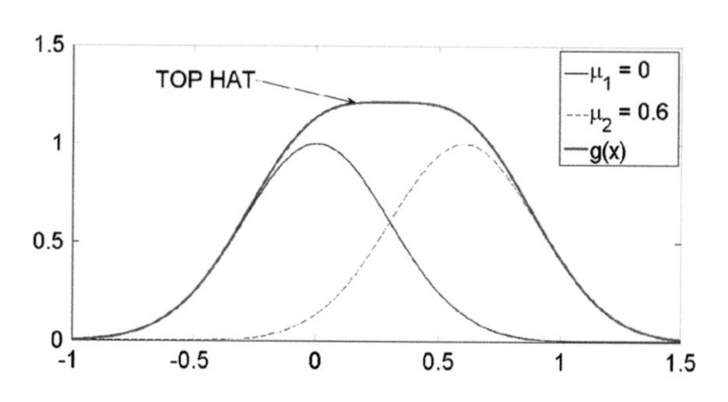

Fig. C.1 Sum of two Gaussians (g(x), *red*) and the values for μ that produce a *top hat* profile

L. Fichera, *Cognitive Supervision for Robot-Assisted Minimally Invasive Laser Surgery*, Springer Theses, DOI 10.1007/978-3-319-30330-7

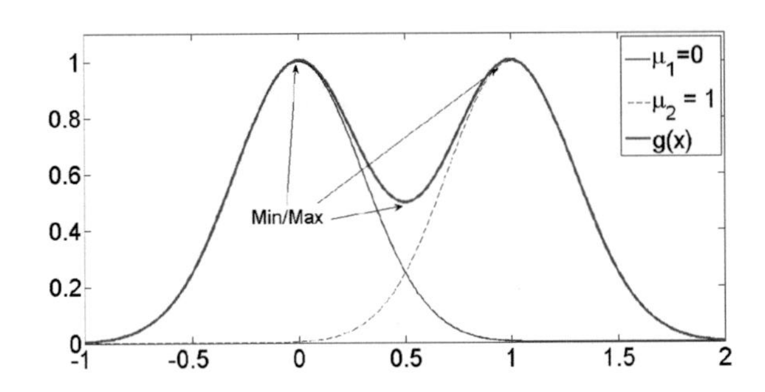

Fig. C.2 Locations where the slope of $g(x)$ is zero (max, min)

The derivative of the equation above,

$$g'(x) = -\frac{ax}{\sigma^2}\exp\left[-\frac{x^2}{2\sigma^2}\right] - \frac{a(x-\mu)}{\sigma^2}\exp\left[-\frac{(x-\mu)^2}{2\sigma^2}\right] \tag{C.4}$$

can be interpreted as the slope of $g(x)$ at any point x of the function domain. Since the top hat is flat, $g'(x)$ must be equal to zero in that region, i.e.

$$x\exp\left[-\frac{x^2}{2\sigma^2}\right] + (x-\mu)\exp\left[-\frac{(x-\mu)^2}{2\sigma^2}\right] = 0. \tag{C.5}$$

It is important to observe that this condition does not depend on the value of the Gaussian amplitude a. For sufficient large values of μ, Eq. C.5 admits at least three solutions, as it can be observed from Fig. C.2.

Let us observe that points in the top hat are located in the range $[0, \mu]$. These can be expressed as a fraction of μ, i.e. $x = \alpha\mu$ for $0 < \alpha < 1$. Replacing $x = \alpha\mu$ and solving for μ in Eq. C.5 yields:

$$\mu = \sqrt{2\sigma^2 \cdot \frac{\log(1-\alpha) - \log(\alpha)}{1-2\alpha}}. \tag{C.6}$$

This relation gives the values of μ for which $g'(\alpha\mu) = 0$. To obtain a top hat profile, we need to ensure that the contribution of the two Gaussians collapse in the middle, i.e. $\alpha \to 1/2$ (Fig. C.3). Equation C.6 is not defined for $\alpha = 5$, thus we need the calculate the limit,

$$\mu_{hat} = \lim_{\alpha\to\frac{1}{2}} \sqrt{2\sigma^2 \cdot \frac{\log(1-\alpha) - \log(\alpha)}{1-2\alpha}}, \tag{C.7}$$

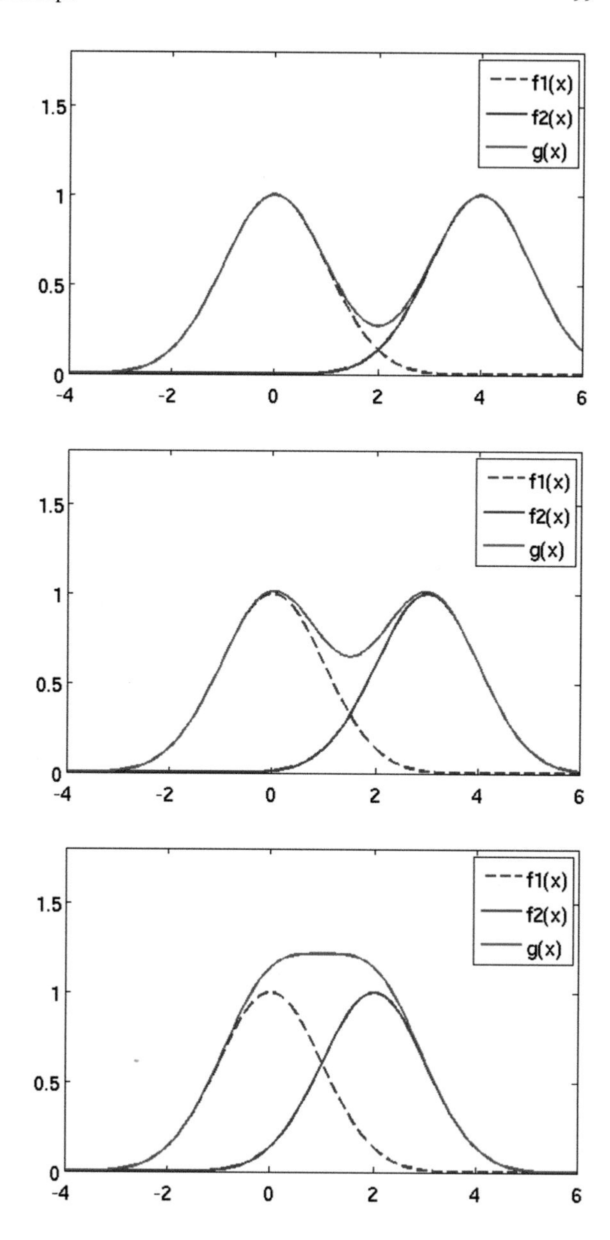

Fig. C.3 Sum of Gaussians for α tending to 1/2

which can be solved applying L'Hôpital's rule:

$$\mu_{hat} = 2 \cdot \sigma \tag{C.8}$$

■